MW00678700

SING TO THE LORD
A NEW SONG

Having had the joy of serving as Gary's associate pastor for six years now, I can honestly say that his life and testimony have served to encourage my walk of faith in so many ways. Gary's life is a shining testament to these glorious promises as he has allowed the power of Christ to give him the strength to overcome severe physical limitations from multiple sclerosis.

—Chuck Patrick, associate pastor,
Silverdale Baptist Church

Many times through the years the Lord has taken me to Psalms to put within me a new song. It is at those times when we are in "the pit" that the Lord will give us a new song. We all face various trials and painful experiences in life, but God never wastes pain. So where do you turn when you face various trials and painful experiences in life? The book of Psalms is where the Lord wants to meet you in your pain and give you a new song of praise.

—S. David Thompson, associate pastor,
Silverdale Baptist Church

JAMES

SING TO THE LORD
A NEW SONG

CELEBRATE   JESUS

Gary Miller . tate Authors . com

gam 2715 @ gmail . com

You to BE : " Modern Day Miracles "

SING TO THE LORD
A NEW SONG

TRANSFORMING LIFE THROUGH SCRIPTURE

GARY MILLER

TATE PUBLISHING & *Enterprises*

Published by Tate Publishing & Enterprises, LLC
127 E. Trade Center Terrace | Mustang, Oklahoma 73064 USA
1.888.361.9473 | www.tatepublishing.com

Tate Publishing is committed to excellence in the publishing industry. The company reflects the philosophy established by the founders, based on Psalm 68:11,
"The Lord gave the word and great was the company of those who published it."

Book design copyright © 2010 by Tate Publishing, LLC. All rights reserved.
Cover design by Blake Brasor
Interior design by Joey Garrett

Published in the United States of America

ISBN: 978-1-61663-335-6
Religion / Devotional
10.08.03

DEDICATION

This book is dedicated to anyone who desires to live and experience life abundantly.

Therefore I urge you, brethren, by the mercies of God, to *present your bodies a living and holy sacrifice,* acceptable to God, which is your spiritual service of worship. And do not be conformed to this world, but *be transformed by the renewing of your mind,* so that you may prove what the will of God is, that which is good and acceptable and perfect.

Romans 12:1–2

The thief comes only to steal and kill and destroy; I came that you might *have life, and have it more abundantly.*

John 10:10

ACKNOWLEDGEMENTS

With a deep humility I stand in awe of all the folks who prayed, encouraged, and supported this book with their time, energy, talents, expertise, and resources. I praise God for who He is and give Him thanks for all of you.

FOREWORD

As a member and deacon of a mega church in Chattanooga, Tennessee, I had received a new family to care for in the deacon ministry. As a fairly new deacon of three years, I was eager to meet and serve our families for whatever their needs where. Gary and Cheryl appeared to be like any other family in our church. But Gary's request was not a common one. He was suffering from progressive multiple sclerosis (MS). He was not very ambulatory at all. His request was that he wanted to do an in-depth Bible study.

I thought, *Great.*

You see, I am an avid participant in discipleship, and this request appealed to me greatly. I was hoping for a study in one of the historical books like Genesis or perhaps a study in one of the major prophetic books or even the book of Revelation. As long as it was not going to be one of the poetic books of the Bible, especially the book of Psalms, I felt okay and well within my comfort zone.

As I prepared to meet with Gary, I somehow sensed what was coming, that *God would not give me what I wanted but what I needed, and that was to "sing to the Lord a new song."* After our first meeting, I proceeded to a Christian bookstore to find a workbook for our study in the book of Psalms. I'll admit that I chose the smallest one I could find. The workbook contained a simple, one-page outline for each of the 150 psalms, and we decided to study each psalm verse by verse, using only footnotes and other reference material found in our Bible.

Gary had recently suffered some serious setbacks in treating his MS when we commenced our study. His doctor had told him to make himself as comfortable as possible, as he had much trouble getting around. I chose our church as a regular place to meet for us because it was very handicap accessible, and I believed that the education building could inspire us to be very studious concerning our lessons. But this turned out not to work well for Gary. The ten-minute trip from his house and the arduous walk, cane in hand, to the classroom was just too much for him. I then suggested we meet in his house, very much like the first-century church members did, in order to minimize the effort on Gary's part. We decided to meet early on Saturday mornings when we were both at our best and study one psalm per week. (The big advantage of doing one-on-one Bible study is that, if it is necessary for one of us to miss a week because of illness or other reasons, the study can readily be picked up where it was left off, unlike group Bible studies where even one absence can cause a participant to miss a key component of the whole study.)

As I knelt before the Lord, he also impressed upon me not to pray for healing for my friend Gary but to continue steadfastly in our study. God placed Acts 2:42 in my consciousness: "And they continued steadfastly in the apostles' doctrine and fellowship, and in breaking of bread, and in prayer."

In addition to our study of doctrine and prayer, we would fellowship over meals, which sometimes included our wives. This convinced me that Gary would improve.

And did he! But I believe that the catalyst for his remission actually involved laying something on the altar of sacrifice; and that was the decision to give up ninety minutes a week for study of doctrine, prayer, and occasionally taking a Saturday to fellowship and break bread together. And, because of grace, we were at liberty when there was a legitimate reason for us to miss an occasional week of study. I saw Gary put down his cane and do things that he never was able to do, like start his own business cleaning ceramic tile floors with a heavy, circular cleaning machine.

Today, Gary sees his MS doctor one time a year. The last time he saw his doctor, he smiled, shook his head, and said, "You're amazing. You are doing better today than when you first were diagnosed."

—John W. Johnson
Gary's discipleship partner

NOTE FROM THE AUTHOR

Sing to the Lord a new song.
Praise Him for who He is.
Give Him thanks for what He has done.

My name is Gary Miller. I surrendered my heart to Jesus January 5, 1969 when I was at a youth retreat. The minister talked about being "saved." I did not understand what that meant. I also heard that Jesus "came to give us life, life more abundant" (John 10:10). I did not know what that meant either. After the service, I talked with a counselor. He explained to me what being "saved" meant. That's when I gave my heart to Jesus. I also asked the counselor what John 10:10 meant. In 1988, nineteen years after surrendering my heart to Jesus, after a series of events, God desires a broken spirit; a broken and contrite heart You will not despise (Psalm 51:17). After striving for nineteen years, God started showing me what John 10:10 meant. I surrendered my heart and life to Jesus. I began a journey in understanding a very basic biblical truth.

Psalm 96:1–8 tells us to *"sing to the Lord a new song."* This truth is a day-by-day experience, and I am learning from the Bible verses talked about all throughout this devotional. I have found that there is *transforming power in praising God for who He is and giving thanks for what He has done.* My life has changed and continues to change—my whole being, perspectives, perceptions, thoughts, attitudes, and behaviors. My life is easier; less stressful; and I am a healthier, happier person emotionally, psychologically, and spiritually. God has allowed me those divine moments to share my faith and what John 10:10 means.

In my younger days, I was an athlete. In 1970, I had major back surgery because of a football injury. I had discs removed and vertebrae fused. I can remember learning to walk all over again. I would have one nurse under one arm and another nurse under the other arm, kicking my legs out in front of me to take a step. I fell to my knees and cried to God, "This is not the abundant life!" In 1979, I had a head injury from playing hockey, which the doctor said resulted in a stroke. My whole left side was numb. At that time, I had to learn to think, walk, and talk all over again. I went through occupational therapy, physical therapy, and speech therapy. I had to learn the elementary ABCs all over again. I had to learn concept matching and identify colors and pictures again. This was at the age of twenty-nine. Again I fell to my knees and cried to God, "This is not the abundant life in my eyes."

I had lost my ability to perform physically on a high competitive level and my ability to perform mentally. I know what it is like when laughter causes physical pain. I have had the experience of feeling the depth of aloneness. I would pick up the phone just to listen to the dial tone to hear that there is a world out there.

In 2002, I was diagnosed with progressive multiple sclerosis (MS):

That diagnosis did not bother me as much as the previous injuries. I praised God for who He is, and I gave Him thanks for what He has done. He has given me His presence, power, strength, mercy, tenderness, and loving kindness day by day to walk with Him. I am healthier emotionally, psychologically, and spiritually. In some ways, God is healing my MS. I am understanding more what each new day means. I am understanding what *John 10:10 means: "I've come that you might have life and have it more abundantly."*

I have tried four different kinds of medications for my MS. None of these medications helped me. I have been medication free since October 2007. My last brain MRI showed my MS has gone into the inactive stage.

When I was diagnosed with progressive MS, I was having a hard time talking. The MS was affecting my vocal cords. My voice was weak, gravely, breaking up, and I did a lot of coughing. Today, my speech is strong and clear. I was using a cane, a walker, and a three-wheel motor cart to get around. Today, I only use a cane occasionally for stability.

God has literally taken me from emptiness to a life full in Jesus.

God has taken me from the depth of aloneness to fullness in Jesus.

God has taken a broken body, healed it, and made me whole in Jesus.

God has taken me from sadness and depression to gladness, joy, peace, contentment, and courage in Jesus.

God has taken me from using a cane, a walker, and a three-wheel scooter to earning money by cleaning ceramic tile floors.

Because He lives, I can face tomorrow.

Sing to the Lord a new song.

Praise God for who He is.

Give Him thanks for what He has done.

A LIFESTYLE OF PRAISING GOD FOR WHO HE IS AND GIVING HIM THANKS FOR WHAT HE HAS DONE

Are you struggling to find joy in life? Are you unable to sing praise to the Lord? As you search each verse in this devotional, underline and write down words that describe who God is, His character and nature, and what He has done.

At the end of each devotion, write down your praise for who God is and your thanks for what He has done. Use the blank pages to write down all the verses that say, "Sing to the Lord a new song," that use the words *praise* and *give thanks*.

Here are a few attributes you could put on your list.

God's nature: He knows all things, sees all things, feels all things, hears all things, and He is everywhere all the time. "God is spirit."

Examples of God's character: rock, shelter, shield, hope, live, truth, way.

Examples of God's work: saves, provides, protects, gives, leads, washes.

As you continue your study also take note of the word *will*. When the Lord says "He will," generally He is stating a *promise*.

Also where the Bible states "God has," this may be a promise.

Make a list of all the promises the Lord makes.

Please note *all* the words that are in *italics* are my emphasis.

> God said, "Let Us make man in Our image, according to Our likeness.
>
> Genesis 1:26

Describe what the image of God looks like in your own words.

_____

_____

_____

Your perceptions and perspectives of who God is, His image, are the deciding factor for your life.

> Therefore if any man is in Christ, he is a *new creature;* old things passed away; *behold, new things have come.*
>
> 2 Corinthians 5:17

Put this verse in your own words.

_____

_____

_____

> Therefore we do not lose heart, but though the outer man is decaying, yet our *inner man is being renewed day by day.*
>
> 2 Corinthians 4:16

In your own words, what does this verse say?
How are we renewed day by day?

_____

_____

> And they, having become callous, having given themselves over to sensuality for the practice of every kind of impurity with greediness. But you did not learn Christ in this way, if indeed you have heard Him and have *been taught in Him just as truth is in Jesus,* that, in reference to your former manner of life, you *lay aside the old self,* which is being corrupted in accordance with the lust of deceit, and that *you be renewed in the spirit of your mind,* and *put on the new self,* which in the likeness of God has been created in righteousness and holiness of truth.
>
> Ephesians 4:19–24

Define the words *new* and *renew* in your own words.

_____

_____

_____

> Therefore I urge you, brethren, by the mercies of God, to *present your bodies a living and holy sacrifice,* acceptable to God, which is your spiritual service of worship. And do not be conformed to this world, but be *transformed by the renewing of your mind,* so that you may prove what the will of God is, that which is good and acceptable and perfect.
>
> Romans 12:1–2

What does this verse mean to you?

_____

_____

_____

What is "good, acceptable, and perfect?"

_____

_____

_____

Work out your salvation with fear and trembling; for it is God who is at work in you, both to will and to work for His good pleasure.

Philippians 2:12

What does it mean to "work out your salvation?"

_____

_____

_____

Be diligent to present yourself approved to God as a workman who does not need to be ashamed, accurately handling the word of truth.

2 Timothy 2:15

What does the word *diligent* mean in relation to this verse?

_____

_____

_____

What does a "workman who does not need to be ashamed" look like to you?

_____

_____

How are we "approved to God?"

_____

_____

_____

I came that you might have life and have it more abundantly.

John 10:10

Sing to the Lord a new song.
Praise God for who He is.
Give Him thanks for what He has done.

Sing for joy in the Lord, O you righteous ones; *praise is becoming to the* upright. *Give thanks to the Lord.* with the lyre; *sing praise to Him* with a harp of ten strings. *Sing to Him a new song;* [play skillfully] with the shout of joy. *For the word of the Lord is upright, And all His work is done in faithfulness. He loves* righteousness and justice; The earth is full of the *loving kindness of the Lord. By the word* of the Lord the heavens were made, *And by the breath* of His mouth all their host. *He gathers* the waters of the sea Together as a heap; *He lays up* the deeps in store houses. Let all the earth fear the Lord; Let all the inhabitants of the world *stand in awe* of Him. For *He spoke* and it was done; *He commanded* and it stood fast. The *Lord nullifies* the counsel of the nations; *He frustrates* the plans of the peoples.

The counsel of the Lord stands forever, the plans of His heart from generation to generation. *Blessed is the nation whose God is the Lord,* The people whom *He has chosen* for His own inheritance. The Lord *looks* from Heaven; *He sees* all the sons of men; From His dwelling place *He looks* out on all the inhabitance of the earth, *He who fashions* the heart of them all, *He who understands* all their works. The king is not saved by a mighty army; A warrior is not delivered by great strength. Behold the *eye of the Lord is on those who fear Him, On those who hope for His loving kindness, To deliver their soul from death And to keep them alive in* famine. Our soul waits for the Lord; *He is our help and our shield.* For our heart rejoices in Him, Because we trust in His *holy name.* Let your loving kindness, O Lord, be upon us, According as *we have hoped in You.*

Psalm 33

To be able to *sing a new song* is a work in progress. It requires a true faith, complete surrender, everlasting trust, and total obedience to the Lord. As I mentioned earlier, my Christian experiences started when I met Jesus in 1969. Being able to *sing a new song* to the Lord was put in gear in 1988. Since then it has been an honor and privilege for me to be able to share the Jesus I am getting to know. He will never leave me or forsake me (Hebrews 13:5).

We can sing a new song. We can praise Him. We can give Him thanks if we don't grow weary and faint (Galatians 6:9).

According to Psalm 33, the characteristics of singing a new song to the Lord are:

1. "Singing with joy"
2. "Being righteous"
3. "Being upright"
4. "Singing praises"
5. "Giving thanks"
6. "Playing skillfully"

How are we able to *sing a new song* to the Lord?
1. Because the "word of the Lord is upright."
2. Because "all of the work of the Lord is done in faithfulness."

In your own words, how can we play skillfully?

List the wonderful works of God in this psalm.

_____

_____

_____

_____

_____

There are at least twenty-four characteristics of God in this scripture. Can you find them? List them.

_____

_____

_____

_____

_____

_____

List all the promises from Psalm 33.

_____

_____

_____

_____

_____

_____

The promise I have experienced is "He is my help."

God has been my sustaining power. When I am weak, He is strong.

"Therefore I am well content with weakness, with insults, with distress, with persecutions, with difficulties, for Christ sake; for when I am weak I am strong" (2 Corinthians 12:10).

For me personally if there is not something going wrong, I have questions.

Jesus is supernatural resurrection power.

> For I consider that the sufferings of this present time are not worthy to be compared with the glory that is to be revealed to us.
>
> Romans 8:18

> And we know that God causes all things to work together for good to those who love God, to those who are called according to His purpose. For those whom He foreknew, He also predestined to be *conformed to the image of His Son,* so that He would be the firstborn among many brethren; and these whom He predestined, He also called; and these whom He called, He also justified; and these whom He justified, He also glorified.
>
> Romans 8:28–30

If we sing to the Lord a new song every day, praising Him for who He is and giving Him thanks for what He has done, we will be in a continuous state of transformation. Are you ready for this experience?

Sing to the Lord a new song.
Praise Him for who He is.
Give Him thanks for what He has done.

> *I waited patiently* for the Lord; And *He inclined to me and heard my cry. He brought me up* out the pit of destruction, out of the miry clay, and He *set my feet upon a rock making my footsteps firm. He put a new song in my mouth, a song of praise To our God;* Many *will see and fear* and will *trust* in the Lord. How *blessed is the man who has made*

the Lord his trust, You, O Lord will not *withhold Your compassion from me; Your loving kindness and truth will continually preserve me.* For evils beyond number have surrounded me; My iniquities have over taken me, so that I am unable to see; They are more numerous than the hairs on my head, and my heart has failed me. Be pleased, O Lord, to *deliver me; Make haste, O Lord, to help me.* Let those be ashamed and humiliated together who seek my life to destroy it; Let those be turned back and dishonored who delight in my hurt. Let those be appalled because of their shame who say to me, "Aha, aha!" Let all who seek You rejoice and be glad in You; Let those who love Your salvation say continually, *"The Lord be magnified!"* Since I am afflicted and needy, let the Lord be mindful of me. You are *my help* and *my deliverer;* do not delay, O my God.

Psalm 40:1–4, 11–17

God's works are done wonderfully.

With God's strength and power, we can do our work, and we can do it wonderfully. Give thought to the characteristics of what *wonderful* looks like to you.

What would be the characteristics of "miry clay?"

_____

_____

_____

_____

Meditate on God's characteristics in pulling us out of the miry clay.

Characteristics such as strength, power, compassion, and tenderness.

Write out your own list of characteristics.

_____

_____

_____

_____

_____

_____

If God places us on a solid rock, wouldn't that make Him a solid rock?

What other characteristics would describe who God is from this psalm?

_____

_____

_____

_____

After we are pulled out of the mud of life and placed on the rock, God will give us confidence and assurance that He will take care of us. We are able to "sing a new song to the Lord."

Write out your thoughts and comments.

_____

_____

_____

_____

What are the characteristics of God in the last verse?

_____

_____

_____

_____

List all the promises in this psalm.

_____

_____

_____

_____

_____

Sing to the Lord a new song.
Praise God for who He is.
Thank God for what He has done.

> *Sing to the Lord a new song; sing to the Lord, all
> the earth. Sing to the Lord, bless His name; proclaim
> good tidings of His salvation from day to day. Tell of
> His glory among all the nations, His wonderful deeds
> among all peoples. For great is the Lord and greatly
> to be praised; He is to be feared above all gods. For all
> the gods of all the peoples are idols, But the Lord made
> the heavens. Splendor and majesty are before Him,
> strength and beauty are in His Sanctuary.*

Psalm 96:1–8

This is a celebration psalm. When we have experienced the "wonderful deeds" and "good tidings"
of His salvation, then we can "sing a new song to
the Lord." Again in this psalm David has experienced God in a supernatural way and has set his
feet on a solid rock. God is protecting David from
evil. He has experienced His power in making
him strong and has set him apart from the foes.

Therefore he is able to "sing a new song to the Lord."

What does it take for us to experience the "wonderful deeds" and "good tidings" of the Lord? Write out your thoughts on this question.

_____

_____

_____

_____

_____

Define *splendor* and *majesty*.
Define *strength* and *beauty*.

We find strength and beauty in the sanctuary of the Lord.

What does this mean?

_____

_____

_____

_____

_____

_____

_____

_____

What are good tidings?

_____

_____

_____

What are the characteristics of God?

_____

_____

_____

Sing to the Lord a new song.
Praise Him for who He is.
Give Him thanks for what He has done.

> *O sing to the Lord a new song, For He has done wonderful things, His right hand and His holy arm have gained the victory for Him.* The Lord *has made known His salvation;* He *has revealed* His righteousness in the sight of the nations. *He has*

remembered His loving kindness and His *faithful-*
ness To the house of Israel; *all the ends of the earth*
have seen the salvation of *our God. Shout joyfully* to
the Lord, all the earth; Break forth and *sing for*
joy and sing praises. Sing praises to the Lord with
the lyre and the sound of melody. With trumpets
and the sound of the horn *shout joyfully* before the
King, the Lord.

Psalm 98:1–6

What is the victory?

How has God "gained the victory?"

_____

_____

_____

_____

How has the Lord "made known His salvation?"

_____

_____

_____

_____

What does it mean: "He will judge the world with righteousness and the people with equity?"

What is "equity," and what kind of "equity" is the Bible referring to?

_____

_____

_____

_____

_____

_____

What are the wonderful things God has done for us?

Sing to the Lord a new song.
Praise God for who He is.
Give Him thanks for what He has done.

> *Blessed be the Lord, my rock , who trains my hands for war,* and my fingers for battle; My *loving kindness* and my *fortress,* my *stronghold* and my *deliverer,* my *shield* and He whom I take *refuge, Who subdues* my people under me. O Lord, what is man, that You take knowledge of him? Or the Son of man, that You think of him? Man is like mere breath; his days are like a passing shadow. *I will sing a new song to You, O God;* upon a harp of ten strings *I will sing praises to You,* Who *gives salvation to*

the kings, Who *rescues* David His servant from the evil sword. *Rescue me and deliver me* out of the hands of aliens, whose mouth speaks deceit and whose right hand is a hand of falsehood.

How blessed are the people who are so situated; how blessed are the people God is the Lord!

Psalm 144

This verse states that the Lord trains our hands for battle. What kind of war is He talking about? This psalm also states that the Lord is my stronghold, rock, fortress, shield, and refuge. If these are some characteristics of God, He will subdue our enemy, rescue us, and deliver us from them. When He does this we are able to "sing a new song to the Lord." What and who are our "enemies?" List at least twelve characteristics of God.

What are the promises in this psalm?

_____

_____

_____

_____

_____

_____

_____

_____

_____

_____

Sing to the Lord a new song.
Praise God for who He is.
Give Him thanks for what He has done.

If God has chosen us, He upholds us, and He delights
in us. He has put His Spirit upon us and has "called us
in righteousness." He has given us a "covenant." What
is the "covenant" God has given us?

_____

_____

_____

_____

_____

God will hold us by the hand and make us a light unto
the nations.
    If God will do these things, how much do you think
He cares for us?
    God has made available to us a lifestyle of "singing
to Him a new song."
    Praise God for who He is.
    Give Him thanks for what He has done.

In this portion of scripture God is showing many of His characteristics. A few of them would be His care for us: compassion, tenderness, grace, and mercy. Make your list of God's characteristics you see here. What are God's promises?

_____

_____

_____

_____

_____

_____

_____

Sing to the Lord a new song.
Praise God for who He is.
Give Him thanks for what He has done.

Then Moses and the sons of Israel sang this song to the Lord, And said; "I will *sing to the Lord,* for *He is highly exulted;* The horse and his rider He has hurled into the sea. *The Lord is my strength and my song,* And *He has become my salvation; this is my God,* And I will *praise Him;* my father's God, and I will *extol Him.* The *Lord is a warrior,* the *Lord is His name.* Your right hand, O Lord, is *majes-*

tic in power, Your right hand, O Lord, shatters the enemy. *And in the greatness of Your excellence You overthrow those who rise up against You: Who is like You among the gods, O Lord? Who is like You, majestic in holiness, awesome in praises, Working wonders? You stretch out Your right hand, The earth swallowed them. In Your loving kindness You have led the people whom You have redeemed; In Your strength You have guided them to Your Holy habitation. The peoples have heard, they tremble;* Terror and dread has fallen upon them; By the greatness of Your arm they are motionless as a stone; Until Your people pass over, O Lord. Until the people pass over whom You have purchased. You will bring them and plant them in the mountains of Your inheritance, The place, O Lord which You have made for Your dwelling, The *sanctuary,* O Lord, which You have established. *The Lord shall reign forever and ever."*

Exodus 15:1–3, 6–7, 11–14, 16–18

Moses says, "this is my God. He has become my salvation. The Lord is a warrior. The Lord is His name." Moses has experienced the "majesty, holiness and excellence" of the Lord. The Lord is "awesome in praise, working wonders." Moses has experienced the Lord's loving kindness, strength, and power. He will "exalt and extol" the Lord. Moses states, "the Lord will reign forever." *We can experience the Lord! We can "sing to the Lord a new song:" a song of praise for who God is and give Him thanks for what He has done.*

What is and what does a sanctuary look like to you?

In this scripture, how is Moses able to testify of God?

What are the characteristics Moses displays in this scripture?

You could start your list with confidence and assurance.

_____

_____

_____

_____

_____

_____

_____

_____

_____

Sing to the Lord a new song.
Praise God for who He is.
Give Him thanks for what He has done.

> Oh *give thanks to the Lord, call upon His name;*
> *Make known His deeds among the peoples. Sing to*
> *Him, Sing praises to Him; Speak of all His wonders.*

Glory to His holy name; Let the heart of those who seek the Lord be glad. Seek the Lord and His strength; Seek His face continually. Remember His *wonderful deeds which He has done, He is the Lord our God; His judgments are in all the earth. Remember His covenant forever, Sing to the Lord, all the earth; Proclaim good tidings of His salvation from day to day. Tell of His glory among the nations, His wonderful deeds among all the peoples.* For great is the Lord and greatly to be praised; He also is to feared above all gods. For all gods of all peoples are idols, *But the Lord made the heavens. Splendor and majesty are before Him, Strength and joy are in His place.* Ascribe to the Lord O families of the peoples, *Ascribe to the Lord glory and strength. Ascribe to the Lord the glory due His name;* Bring an offering, and come before Him; Worship the Lord in holy array. Tremble before Him, all the earth; Indeed the world is firmly established, it will not be moved. *Let the heavens be glad,* and *let the earth rejoice;* And let them say among the nations, *"the Lord reigns!"* Let the sea roar, and all it contains; Let the field exult, and all that is in it. Then the trees of the forest will sing for joy before the Lord; For He is coming to judge the earth. O *give thanks* to the Lord, for He is good; For His loving kindness is *everlasting.* Then say, *"save us, O God of our salvation,* And *gather us* and *deliver us* from the nations, *To give thanks to Your holy name, And Glory in your Praise."* Blessed be the Lord, the God of Israel, From everlasting to everlasting. Then all the people said "amen," and praised the Lord!

1 Chronicles 16:8–12, 14–15, 23–36

If we seek the Lord and His strength and seek the His face continually, we will find "splendor and majesty, strength and joy." Then we will be able to "Sing to the Lord a new song." We will be able to tell of His wonderful works and give Him praise for who He is and thanks for what He has done.

What are the characteristics of the Lord listed here?

_____

_____

_____

In your own words what does God's loving kindness look like?

_____

_____

_____

Sing to the Lord a new song.
Praise God for who He is.
Give Him thanks for what He has done.

> O Lord, You have searched me and known me. *You know* when I sit down and when I rise up; *You understand* my thoughts from afar. *You scrutinize my path* and my laying down, And are *intimately acquainted* with all my ways. Even before

there is a word on my tongue, behold, O Lord, You *know it all.* You have *enclosed me* behind and before, And *laid Your hand upon me. Such* knowledge is too wonderful for me; It is too high, I cannot attain it. Where can I go from Your Spirit? Or where can I flee from Your presence? If I ascend to heaven, You are there; If I make my bed in SHEOL, behold, You are there. If I take the wings of the dawn, If I dwell in the remotest part of the sea, Even there *Your hand will lead me.* If I say, "surely the darkness overwhelms me, And the light about me will be night," Even the darkness is not dark to You, And the night is as bright as the day. Darkness and light are alike to You. *For You formed my inward parts; You wove me in my mother's womb. I will give thanks to You, for I am fearfully and wonderfully made; Wonderful are Your works, And my soul knows it very well. My frame was not hidden from You, When I was made in secret, And skillfully wrought in the depths of the earth;* Your eyes have seen my unformed substance; And *in Your book were all written The days You ordained for me,* When as yet there was not one of them. How *precious also are Your thoughts to me,* O God! How vast is the sum of them! If I should count them, they would outnumber the sand. When I awake, I am still with You.

Psalm 139:1–18

God created man. He knows his ways, his days. God knows everything about us. God allows things in our life to make us the kind of beings He desires us to be for eternal purposes. In my own life He has allowed things to happen to make me a better person from a spiritual perspective. God has allowed physical pain, mental anguish, and psychological stress so that I would be more true in my faith, more dependent on Him, and more trusting of Him. God *never* has failed nor let me down! Romans 8:28: "God causes *all* things to work together for good to those who love God, to those who are called according to His purpose." Romans 8:18: "for I consider that the suffering of this present time are not worthy to be compared with the glory that is to be revealed to us." What a promise. List other promises you see in this psalm.

List words that describe God's character.

_____

_____

_____

Examine your life. With true faith, complete surrender, total obedience, and everlasting trust, can you see how God is making you into the person He wants you to be?

Share your thoughts of how you see God constructing your life for *His* purpose.

_____

_____

_____

Sing to the Lord a new song.
Praise God for who He is.
Give Him thanks for what He has done.

> O Lord, our Lord, *How majestic* is *Your name* in all the earth, Who have *displayed Your splendor* above the heavens! From the mouth of infants and nursing babes You *have Established strength* Because of Your adversaries, to make the enemy and the revengeful cease. When I consider Your heavens, the work of Your fingers, The moon and the stars, which You *have ordained:* What is man that You take thought of him, and the son of man that You care for him? Yet You have *made him a little lower than God, And you crown him with glory and majesty!* You make him to rule over the works of Your hands;
>
> Psalm 8:1–6

In this psalm we see an emphasis placed on God's sovereignty; "your name" refers to the revealed person of who God is and all of His character. God is majestic in splendor and strength.

O Lord, my Lord, Your majesty and splendor reach far above the heavens. Because of Your great strength and power, we are able to experience You in our innermost being and able to sing to You a "new song." We will praise You for who You are and give You thanks for Your wonderful works.

Sing to the Lord a new song.
Praise God for who He is.
Give Him thanks for what He has done.

I will give thanks to the Lord with all my heart: *I will tell* of Your wonders. *I will be glad and exult in You; I will sing praises to Your name,* O Most High. The enemy has come to an end in perpetual ruins, And You have uprooted the cities; The very memory of them has perished. But *the Lord abides forever;* He has established His throne for judgment, And He will judge the world in *righteousness; He will execute judgment for the people with equity. The Lord will also be a stronghold for the oppressed, A stronghold in the times of trouble; And those who know Your name will put their trust in You. For You, O Lord, have not forsaken those who seek You. Sing praises to the Lord,* who dwells in ZION; declare among the people His deeds. He does not forget the cry of the afflicted. Be gracious to me, O Lord; See my affliction from those who hate me, *You who lifted me up* from the gates of death, That I may tell of all Your praises, That in the gates of the daughter of Zion I may rejoice in Your salvation.

Psalm 9:1–2, 6–14

Once you have experienced the Lord and His strength and power to overcome "the mud" of this life, and found Him to be a stronghold, you will want to declare the Lord as true and trusting. In dealing with my MS, I have found a strength, a power, a peace, and a presence that only can come from the Lord.

He has given me a "new song" to sing and a reason

to do that. I can praise God for who He is and give Him thanks for what He has done.

Sing to the Lord a new song.
Praise God for who He is.
Give Him thanks for what He has done.

O Lord, who may abide in Your tent? Who may dwell on Your holy hill? *He who walks with integrity,* and *works righteousness,* And *speaks truth* in his heart. He does not slander with his tongue, Nor does evil to his neighbor, Nor takes reproach against a friend; In whose eyes a reprobate is despised, *But honors those who fear the Lord;* He swears to his own hurt and does not change; He does not put out his money at interest, Nor does he take a bribe against the innocent. *He who does these things will never be shaken.*

Psalm 15

When we walk with integrity in our heart and honor the Lord in what we say and do, we will never be shaken. God gives us His power, presence, and peace in singing to the Lord a "new song." We are able to praise Him for who He is and give Him thanks for what He has done.

Sing to the Lord a new song.
Praise God for who He is.
Give Him thanks for what He has done.

"I love you, O Lord, my strength." The Lord is my rock and my fortress and my deliverer, My God, my rock, in whom I take refuge; My shield and the horn

of my salvation, My stronghold. I call upon the Lord, who is worthy to be praised, And *I am saved* from my enemies. The cords of death encompassed me, And the torrents of the ungodly terrified me. The cords of SHEOL surrounded me; The snares of death confronted me. In my distress I called upon the Lord, And cried to my God for help; *He heard* my voice out of His temple, And my cry for help; before Him came into His ears. At your rebuke, O Lord, At the blast of the breath of Your nostrils. He sent from on high, *He took me; He drew me out* of many waters. *He delivered me* from my strong enemy, And from those who hated me. For they were to mighty for me. They confronted me in the day of my calamity, *But the Lord was my stay. He brought me forth also into a broad place; He rescued me, because He delighted in me. The Lord has rewarded me according to my righteousness; According to the cleanness of my hands, He has recompensed me. For I have kept the ways of the Lord, And have not wickedly departed from my God. For all His ordinances were before me, And I did not put away His statutes from me. I was also blameless with Him, And I have kept myself from my iniquity. Therefore the Lord has recompensed me according to my righteousness, According to the cleanness of my hands in His eyes.* With the kind, You show *Yourself kind;* With the blameless You show *Yourself blameless;* With the *pure You show Yourself pure,* And with the crooked You show Yourself astute. *For You save the afflicted people,* But haughty eyes You abase. For *You light my lamp; my God illumines my darkness.* For *by You I can run* upon a troop; And by *my God I can leap over a wall. As for God, His way is blameless; the word of the Lord is tried; He is a* shield to all those who take refuge in Him. *For who is God but the Lord? And who is a rock except our God. The God who girds me with strength and makes my way blameless? He makes my feet like hinds feet, And sets me upon high places. He trains my hands for battle, So that my arms can bend a bow of bronze. You have also given me the shield of Your salvation, And Your right hand upholds me; And Your gentleness makes me great. You enlarge my steps under me, And my feet have not slipped.* I pursued my enemies and overtook them, And I did not turn back until they were consumed. I shattered them, so that they were not able to rise; They fell under my feet. *For You have girded me with strength* for battle; You have subdued under me those who rose up against me. You have also made my enemies turn their backs to me, And I destroyed those who hated me. They cried for help, but there was none to save, Even to the Lord, but He did not answer them. Then I beat them fine as the dust before the wind; I emptied them out as mire of the streets. *You have delivered me from the contentions of the people;* You have placed me as the head of the nations; A people I have not known serve me. As soon as they hear, they obey me; Foreigners submit to me. Foreigners fade away, And come trembling out of their fortress. *The Lord lives and blessed be my rock; And exalted be the God of my salvation, The God who executes vengeance for me, And subdues peoples under me. He delivers me from my enemies; Surely You lift me above those who rise up against me; You rescue me from the violent man.* Therefore *I will give thanks to You* among the nations, O Lord, And I will *sing praises to Your name. He gives great deliverance* to the king, And shows loving kindness to His anointed, To David and his descendants forever.

Psalm 18:1–6, 15–50

In this psalm we see the caring compassion of God with His outstretched hand of tenderness who intimately knows all of our ways. He understands our issues in life, carries us through our issues, delivers us from them, and raises us to a firm foundation in Jesus. Once God sets us on that firm foundation, He "recompenses" us according to our righteousness. God will rescue us because He delights in us. What does the phrase "He delights in us" mean?

_____

_____

_____

_____

_____

God performs His mighty works in us and through us so that we are a light unto the nations so that they can see His testimonies are true and lasting forevermore.

God desires us to be a true testimony unto Him.

Romans 9:17: "I raised you up to demonstrate My power in you, and that My name be proclaimed throughout the whole earth."

There are over seventy-five words in this psalm that describe God's nature, His character and what He has done for us. List them.

_____

_____

_____

Sing to the Lord a new song.
Praise God for who He is.
Give Him thanks for what He has done.

The heavens are telling the glory of God; And their expanse the work of His hands. *The law of the Lord is perfect, restoring the soul; The testimony of the Lord is sure, making wise the simple. The precepts of the Lord are right, rejoicing the heart; The commandment of the Lord is pure, enlightening the eyes. The fear of the Lord is clean; enduring forever; The judgments of the Lord are true; They are righteous altogether.* They are more desirable than gold, Yes, than much fine gold; sweater also than honey and the drippings of honeycomb. Moreover, by them Your servant is warned; In keeping them, there is great reward. Who can discern his errors? Acquit me of hidden faults. Also keep back Your servant from presumptuous sins; Let them not rule over me; Then I will be blameless. And I shall be acquitted of great transgression. Let the words of my mouth and the meditation of my heart be acceptable in Your sight, *O Lord, my rock and my redeemer.*

The law of the Lord is_____, _____
the soul.
The testimony of the Lord is _____, _____
the simple.
The precepts of the Lord are _____,
_____the heart.
The commandment of the Lord is _____,
_____the eyes.
The fear of the Lord is _____;
_____forever.
The judgments of the Lord are _____; they
are _____.

Psalm 19:1, 7–14

What are the characteristics of the Lord in this psalm?

_____

_____

_____

Sing to the Lord a new song.
Praise God for who He is.
Give Him thanks for what He has done.

O Lord, *in Your strength* the king will be glad,
And *in Your salvation* how greatly he will rejoice!
You *have given* him his heart's desire, And You
have not withheld the request of his lips. *For You
meet him with the blessing of good things; You set a
crown of fine gold on his head. He asked life of You,
You gave it to him, Length of days forever and ever.
His glory is great through Your salvation, Splendor*

*and majesty You place upon him. For You make him
most blessed forever; You make him joyful* with gladness in Your presence.

Psalm 21:1–6

God gives us what we need to be able to greatly
rejoice. He has given us His Son and His character
through the Holy Spirit. Again as we appropriate true
faith, total surrender, complete obedience, and an everlasting trust, God will carry us through life and bring
us out on the other side of all our situations with our
hands raised in victory!

List the promises of God in this psalm.

_____

_____

_____

Sing to the Lord a new song.
Praise God for who He is.
Give Him thanks for what He has done.

The Lord is my shepherd, I shall not want. He *makes
me* lie down in green pastures; *He leads* me beside
quiet waters. *He restores* my soul; *He guides* me in
the paths of righteousness For His name's sake.
Even though I walk through the valley of the
shadow of death, I fear no evil, for You are with
me. Your *rod* and Your *staff,* they comfort me. You
have anointed my head with oil; My cup overflows.
Surely goodness and loving kindness will follow

me all the days of my life, And I will dwell in the
house of the Lord forever.

Psalm 23

A shepherd is a leader, one who herds and takes
care of someone or something, i.e., sheep. Here
God refers to Himself as a shepherd. He takes
care of His people. He guides, directs, protects,
and guards His people. He makes us lie down
by quiet waters. God makes us lie down as He
allows something in our life for a growth process
to take place. If He does this, He will give us the
strength, power, grace, and mercy to endure. His
rod is used for protection against harm. The staff
is used to help in a situation of defense or offense.
The Lord's goodness and mercy will carry us all
the days of our life.

List at least ten characteristics of what He has done
for us.

_____

_____

_____

In your own words, what is the " goodness" of the Lord?

What does *mercy* mean?

_____

_____

_____

_____

_____

List the promises from psalm 23.

_____

_____

_____

_____

Sing to the Lord a new song.
Praise God for who He is.
Give Him thanks for what He has done for us.

The Lord is the Light of my salvation; Whom shall I fear? *The Lord is the defense of my life;* Whom shall I dread? When evildoers came upon me to devour my flesh, My adversaries and my enemies, they stumbled and fell. Though a host encamp against me, My heart will not fear; Though war rise up against me, In spite of this I *shall be confident. One thing I have asked from the Lord, that I shall seek: That I may dwell in the house of the Lord all the days of my life, To behold the beauty of the Lord And to meditate in His temple.* For *in the day of trouble He will conceal me* in His tabernacle; In the secret place of His tent He will *hide me;* He will *lift me up* on a rock. And now my *head will be lifted* above my enemies around me, *And I will offer in His tent sacrifices with shouts of joy; I will sing, yes, I will sing praises to the Lord.* "Hear, O Lord, when I cry with my voice, And be gracious to me and answer me. When You said, 'seek my face,' my heart said to You, Your face, O Lord, I shall seek.' Do not hide Your face from me, Do not turn your servant away in anger; You *have been my help;* Do not abandon me nor forsake me, *O God of my salvation!* For my father and my mother have forsaken me, But the Lord *will take me up. Teach me* Your way, O Lord, And *lead me* in a level path Because of my foes. I would have despaired unless I had believed that I would see the goodness of the Lord in the land of the living." *Wait for the Lord; Be strong and let your heart take courage; Yes, wait for the Lord.*

Psalm 27:1–11, 13–14

List more than twelve characteristics that describe what God has done for us in this psalm.

_____

_____

_____

Sing to the Lord a new song.
Praise God for who He is.
Give Him thanks for what He has done.

I will extol you, O Lord, for You have *lifted me up,*

And have not let my enemies rejoice over me. O Lord my God, I cried to You for help, and You *healed me.* O Lord, You *have brought* up my soul from SHEOL, You have *kept me alive,* that I would not go down to the pit. *Sing praise to the Lord,* you His Godly ones, And *give thanks to His holy name.* For His anger is but for a moment, *His favor is for a lifetime;* Weeping my last for the night; *But a shout of joy comes in the morning.* Now as for me, I said in my prosperity, "I will never be moved." *O Lord, by Your favor You have made my mountain to stand strong;* You hid Your face, I was dismayed. To You, O Lord, I called, And to the Lord I made supplication. Hear, O Lord, and be gracious to me; O Lord, be my *helper. You have turned for me my mourning into dancing; You have loosed my sackcloth and girded me with gladness, That my soul may sing praise to You and not be silent. O Lord my God, I will give thanks to You forever.*

Psalm 30:1–8, 10–12

God is in the transformation business. He is the healer of the soul, mind, and body. He will lift you up out of your pit in life, and He will keep you alive. He will loosen your sackcloth and turn your mourning into dancing. He is our helper and will give us the ability to stand strong. When we have experienced the supernatural resurrection power of Jesus, we can "extol" His name, give thanks, and sing praise to Him for who He is and thank Him for what He has done in our life.

List the promises of the Lord in this psalm.

_____

_____

_____

_____

Sing to the Lord a new song.
Praise God for who He is.
Give Him thanks for what He has done.

I will bless the Lord at all times; His praise shall continually be in my mouth. My soul will make its boast in the Lord; The humble will hear it and rejoice. O magnify the Lord with me, And let us exalt His name together. I sought the Lord, and He *answered me,* And *delivered me* from all my fears. They *looked to Him and were radiant,* And their faces will never be ashamed. *This poor man cried, and the Lord heard him, And saved him out of all his troubles. The angel of the Lord encamps around those who fear Him, and rescues them.* O taste and see that the Lord is good; *How blessed is the man who takes refuge in Him!* O fear the Lord you His saints; *For to those who fear Him there is no want.* The young lions do lack and suffer hunger; But they who seek the Lord shall not be in want of any good thing. Come, you children, listen to Me; I will teach you the fear of the Lord. The face of the Lord is against evildoers, To cut off the memory of them from the earth. *The righteous cry, and the Lord hears And delivers them out of all their troubles. The Lord is near to the broken hearted And saves those who are crushed in spirit. Many are the afflic-*

tions of the righteous, But the Lord delivers him out of them all. He keeps all his bones, not one of them is broken. Evil shall slay the wicked, And those who hate the righteous will be condemned. *The Lord redeems the soul of His servants, And none of those who take refuge in Him will be condemned.*

Psalm 34:1–11, 16–22

There are more than eighteen characteristics of God's nature and character listed in this psalm. Can you list them?

_____

_____

_____

_____

_____

_____

Sing to the Lord a new song.
Praise God for who He is.
Give Him thanks for what He has done for us.

Do not fret because of evil doers, Be *not envious* toward wrongdoers. For they will wither quickly like the grass And fade like the green herb. *Trust in the Lord and do good; Dwell in the land and cultivate faithfulness. Delight yourself in the Lord;* And

He will give you the desires of your heart. *Commit your way to the Lord, trust also in Him,* and He will do it. He will bring forth your righteousness as the light. And your judgment as the noonday. *Rest in the Lord and wait patiently for Him; Do not fret* because of him who prospers in his way, Because of the man who carries out wicked schemes. Cease from anger and forsake wrath; Do not fret; it leads only to evil doing. For evil doers will be cut off, *But those who wait for the Lord, they will inherit the land.* But the humble will inherit the land and will delight themselves in abundant prosperity. The wicked plots against the righteous and gnashes at him with his teeth. The *Lord laughs* at him, For He sees his day is coming. Better is the little of the righteous than the abundance of many wicked, For the arms of the wicked will be broken, But *the Lord sustains the righteous. The Lord knows the days of the blameless, And their inheritance will be forever. They will not be ashamed in the time of evil,* And in the days of famine they will have abundance. But the wicked will perish; and the enemies of the Lord will be like the glory of the pasture, They vanish—like the smoke they vanish away. The wicked borrows and does not pay back, But the righteous is gracious and gives. For those blessed by Him will inherit the land, But those cursed by Him will be cut off. The *steps of a man are established by the Lord, And He delights in his way. When he falls he will not be hurled headlong, Because the Lord is the one who holds his hand. I have been young and now I am old, Yet I have not seen the righteous forsaken. Or his descendants begging for bread. All day long he is gracious and lends, And his descendants are a blessing. Depart from evil and do good, So you will abide forever. For the Lord loves justice, and does not forsake His godly ones. They are preserved forever,* But the descendants of the wicked will be cut off. The righteous will inherit the land And dwell in it forever. The mouth of the righteous utters wisdom, And his tongue speaks justice. *The Law of his God is in his heart; his steps do not slip.* The wicked spies upon the righteous And seeks to kill him. The *Lord will not leave him in his hand or let him be condemned when he is* judged. Wait for the Lord and keep His way, And He will exalt you to inherit the land; When the wicked are cut off, you will see it. Mark the blameless man, and behold the upright; For the man of peace will have posterity. But transgressors will be altogether destroyed; The posterity of the wicked will be cut off. But the *salvation of the righteous is from the Lord; He is their strength in the time of trouble. The Lord helps them and delivers them; He delivers them from the wicked and saves them, Because they take refuge in Him.*

Psalm 37:1–9, 11–13, 16–34, 37–40

When we delight in the Lord, trust in Him, and commit our way to Him, we can have life with no fear from evildoers. We have the power to "live in the land and cultivate faithfulness." When we do this in true faith, complete surrender, total obedience, and an everlasting trust, He will bring forth the desire of his Heart. If we wait patiently for the Lord and rest in Him, He will be exalted in us and through us, and we will "inherit the land." Our steps and our way are designed by the Lord, and if we walk by His ways He will deliver and save us from our enemy.

List all the promises from this psalm.

_____

_____

_____

_____

_____

_____

_____

_____

What does it mean to delight yourself in the Lord?

_____

_____

Sing to the Lord a new song.
Praise God for who He is.
Give Him thanks for what He has done.

> *God is our refuge and strength, A very present help
> in the time of trouble.* Therefore we will not fear,
> though the earth should change And though the
> mountains slip into the sea; Though its waters
> roar and foam, Though the mountains quake at
> its swelling pride. *There is a river whose streams*

*make glad the city of God, The holy dwelling place of
the Most High. God is in the midst of her, she will not
be moved; God will help her when morning dawns.*
Come behold the works of the Lord, Who has
wrought desolations in the earth. He makes wars
cease to the end of the earth; He breaks the bow
and cuts the spear in two; He burns the chariots
with fire. "*Cease striving and know that I am God;
I will be exalted among the nations, I will be exalted
in the earth.*" *The Lord of host is with us; The God of
Jacob is our stronghold.*

Psalm 46:1–5, 8–11

Because God is our refuge, strength, help, and
stronghold, why should we live in fear?

As I stated earlier, I made a heart surrender to Jesus
in 1969. In 1970 I had major back surgery. It took a
long time to be active again. I spent more time lying
flat. During therapy I had to learn to walk. I was made
to be "still and quiet." I fought this whole time and
process. In 1976 I was in the hospital for seven weeks in
traction. Again I fought this whole time of being still
and quiet.

Psalm 23:2: "God makes us lie down in green pastures." There is a purpose in being quiet and still.

In 1979 I had a head injury, which resulted in a
stroke. My whole left side was paralyzed. I went
through physical therapy, speech therapy, and occupational therapy. I was made to be quiet and still. It was
at this time I started to learn Psalm 46:10: "be still and
know that I am God."

In 1998 I had more back surgery. In the same year I
had both rotator cuffs surgically repaired.

In 2002 I was diagnosed with MS; the hot weather

really bothers me. I cannot be outside during hot days. I have more pain from my MS with cold weather. When it is cold and raining, I can hardly get out of bed. Again I am made to be quiet and still.

That process does not bother me anymore as I have learned the meaning and purpose of being quiet and still. God gives us the times of being quiet and still to teach us and build our character. "Cease striving and know that He is God!"

Can you list reasons why we are made to "be still and know I am God?"

One reason might be for refreshment for the mind, body, and soul.

_____

_____

_____

_____

_____

_____

Sing to the Lord a new song.
Praise God for who He is.
Give Him thanks for what He has done.

Clap your hands, all peoples; shout to God with the voice of joy. For the Lord Most High is to be feared, A great King over all the earth. He subdues peoples under us And nations under our feet. He chooses our inheritance for us, Sing praises to God, sing praises; Sing praises to our King, sing praises. For God is the King of all the earth; Sing praises with a skillful psalm. God reigns over all the nations, God sits on His holy throne.

Psalm 47:1–4, 6–8

List more than seven characteristics of God from this psalm.

_____

_____

_____

Sing to the Lord a new song.
Praise God for who He is.
Give Him thanks for what He has done.

O God, you are my God; I shall seek You earnestly; My soul thirst for You, my flesh yearns for You, in a dry and weary land where there is no water. Thus I have seen You in the sanctuary. To see Your power and Your glory. Because Your loving kindness is better than life, My lips will praise you. So I will bless You as long as I live; I will lift up my hands in Your name. My soul is satisfied as with marrow and fatness, And my mouth offers praises with joyful lips. When I remember You on my bed, I meditate on You in the night watches,

For You have been my help, And in the shadow of Your wings I sing for joy. My soul clings to You; Your right hand upholds me.

Psalm 63:1–8

When we seek the Lord with a true faith and proper heart attitude, we are able to see the Lord in all of His glory, splendor, and majesty. Then our soul is satisfied, and we can praise Him for who He is and give Him thanks for what He has done! We can sing to the Lord a "new song."

List the characteristics of God in this psalm.

_____

_____

_____

Sing to the Lord a new song.
Praise God for who He is.
Give Him thanks for what He has done.

Shout joyfully to God, all the earth; sing the glory of His name; Make His Praise glorious. say to God, "how awesome are Your works! Because of the greatness of Your power Your enemies will give feigned obedience to You. All the earth will worship You, And will sing praises to You; They will sing praises to Your name." *Come and see the works of God, Who is awesome in His deeds toward the sons of men.* Come and hear, all who fear God, And I will tell of what He has done for my soul. I cried to Him with my mouth And He was extolled with my tongue. If I regard wickedness in my heart, The Lord will not hear; But certainly God has heard, He has given heed to the voice of my prayer. *Blessed be God Who has not turned away my prayer, Nor His loving kindness from me.*

Psalm 66:1–5, 16–20

When we fall to our knees and cry to the Lord in true humility of a broken spirit, emotionally, psychologically, and physically, God will hear our voice and cover us with His loving kindness. We can shout joyfully, singing glory to His name.

List more than ten characteristics of God from this psalm.

List the promises of the Lord in the psalm.

Sing to the Lord a new song.
Praise God for who He is.
Give Him thanks for what He has done.

> How lovely are Your dwelling places, O Lord of hosts! My soul longed and even yearned for the courts of the Lord; My heart and my flesh sing for joy to the living God. *They go from strength to strength,* Every one of them appears before God in Zion. O Lord God of hosts, hear my prayer; Give ear, O God of Jacob! Behold our shield, O God, And look upon the face of your anointed. *For a day in Your courts is better than a thousand outside.* I would rather stand at the threshold of the house of my God Than to dwell in the tents of wickedness. *For the Lord God is a sun and a shield; The Lord gives grace and glory; no good thing does He withhold from those who walk uprightly. O Lord of hosts, how blessed is the man who trusts in You!*
>
> Palm 84:1–2, 7–12

When we dwell where the Lord is, we will find strength and power and see the Lord for who He is. Then we are able to bless the Lord, praise the Lord, and give Him praise for who He is and thanks for what He has done.

Where is the Lord?

_____

_____

_____

_____

_____

_____

Sing to the Lord a new song.
Praise God for who He is.
Give Him thanks for what He has done.

> *He who dwells in the shelter* of the Most High *Will abide* in the shadow of the Almighty. I will say to the Lord, "*my refuge and my fortress; My God* in whom I trust!" For it is *He who delivers you* from the snare of the trapper And from the deadly pestilence. *He will* cover you with His pinions, And *under His wings you may seek refuge;* His faithfulness is a shield and a bulwark. *You will not be afraid* of the terror by night, Or the arrow that flies by the day; Of the pestilence that stalks in darkness, Or of the destruction that lays waste at noon. A thousand may fall at your side and Ten thousand at your right hand, *But it shall not approach* you. You will only look on with your eyes And see the recompense of the wicked. *For You have made the Lord, my refuge, Even the Most High, Your dwelling place. No evil will befall you, Nor will any plague come near your tent. For He will give His angels charge concerning you, To guard you in all your ways. Because He has loved me, therefore I will deliver him. I will set him securely on high, because he has known My name. He will call upon Me, and I will answer him; I will be with him in trouble; I will rescue him*

and honor him. "with a long life I will satisfy him
And let him see My salvation."

Psalm 91:1–11, 14–16

Count how many times the word "will" is mentioned in the psalm.

List all the promises of the Lord from this psalm.

List the characteristics that define the "name" of the Lord.

_____

_____

_____

_____

_____

_____

List more than fifteen characteristics of the Lord from this psalm.

_____

_____

_____

_____

_____

_____

Sing to the Lord a new song.
Praise God for who He is.
Give Him thanks for what He has done.

> *It is good to give thanks to the Lord, And to sing praises to Your name, O Most High; To declare Your loving kindness in the morning And Your faithfulness by night,* With the ten stringed lute and with the harp, With resounding music upon the lyre. *For You, O Lord, have made me glad by what You have done, I will sing for joy at the works of Your hands. How great are Your works, O Lord! Your thoughts are very deep. A senseless man has no knowledge,* Nor does a stupid man understand this; That when the wicked sprouted up like grass And all who did iniquity flourished, it was only that they might be destroyed forevermore. But You, O Lord, are on high forever. The righteous man will flourish like the palm tree, He will grow like the cedar in Lebanon planted in the house of the Lord, They will flourish in the courts of our God. They will still yield fruit in old age; They shall be full of sap and very green. *To declare that the Lord is upright; He is my rock, and there is no unrighteousness in Him.*
>
> Psalm 92:1–8, 12–15

We are able to give thanks, sing praises, declare His loving kindness, and tell His wonderful works. We will flourish and be glad in the Lord. The Lord is upright. He is and will be my rock!

Sing to the Lord a new song.
Praise God for who He is.
Give Him thanks for what He has done.

> *The Lord reigns, He is clothed with majesty; The Lord has clothed and girded Himself with strength; Indeed, the world is firmly established, it will not be moved. Your throne is established from of old;* You are from everlasting. *The Lord on high is mighty, Your testimonies are fully confirmed; Holiness befits Your house, O Lord, forevermore.*

Psalm 93:1–2, 4–5

List all the promises of the Lord from this psalm.

_____

_____

_____

_____

_____

List more than ten characteristics of the Lord from this psalm.

_____

_____

Sing to the Lord a new song.
Praise God for who He is.
Give Him thanks for He has done.

> *O come, let us sing for joy to the Lord, Let us shout joyfully to the rock of our salvation. Let us come before His presence with thanksgiving, Let us shout joyfully to Him with psalms. For the Lord is a great God and a great* King above all gods, In whose hands are the depths of the earth, The peaks of the mountains are His also, The sea is His, for it was He who made it, And His hands formed the dry land. *Come, let us worship and bow down, Let us kneel before the Lord our maker. For He is our God, And we are the people of His pasture and the sheep of His hand.*

Psalm 95: 1–7

When we bow down and worship the Lord we will find a peace, presence and power only He can give. Then we can "sing for joy to the Lord," and "shout joyfully to the rock of our salvation."

Sing to the Lord a new song.
Praise God for who He is.
Give Him thanks for what He has done for us.

> *Shout joyfully to the Lord, all the earth. Serve the Lord with gladness: Come before Him with joyful singing. Know that the Lord Himself is God: It is He who has made us, and not we ourselves. We are His people and the sheep of His pasture. Enter His gates with thanksgiving and His courts with praise.*

Give thanks to Him, bless His name. For the Lord is good; His loving kindness is everlasting And His faithfulness to all generations.

Psalm 100

Once we have experienced the goodness, loving kindness, and faithfulness of the Lord, we will have the desire to shout and sing of the works of the Lord.

Sing to the Lord a new song.
Praise God for who He is.
Give Him thanks for what He has done.

I will sing of loving kindness and justice to you, O Lord, I will sing Praises. *I will walk within my house in the integrity of my heart. I will set no* worthless thing before my eyes; I *hate the work* of those who fall away; It shall not fasten its grip on me. *A perverse heart* shall depart from me; I will know no evil. Whoever *secretly slanders* his neighbor, *him I will destroy; No one who has a haughty look and an arrogant heart will I endure. My eyes shall be upon the faithful* of the land, That they may dwell with Me; *He who walks in a blameless way is the one who will minister to Me.* He who *practices deceit* shall not dwell within My house; *He who speaks falsehood* shall not maintain his position before Me. Every morning I will destroy all the wicked of the land, So as to cut off from the city of the Lord all those who do iniquity.

Psalm 101

If we walk with integrity in our heart, He will guard us and protect us from evil.

List the promises from this psalm.

_____

_____

_____

_____

_____

_____

_____

_____

List the characteristics of the word *integrity*.

Sing to the Lord a new song.
Praise God for who He is.
Give Him thanks for what He has done.

> *Bless the Lord,* O my soul, And all that is within
> me, *bless* His *holy name. Bless the Lord,* O my soul,
> and *forget none* of His benefits; Who *pardons* all
> of our iniquities, *Who heals* all your diseases; *Who
> redeems* your life from the pit, *Who crowns* you with
> loving kindness and compassion; *Who satisfies*
> your years with good things, So that *your youth is
> renewed like the eagle.* The *Lord performs* righteous

deeds and judgments for all who are oppressed. He *made known* His ways to Moses, *His acts* to the sons of Israel. *The Lord is compassionate and gracious, slow to anger abounding in loving kindness.* He will not always strive with us, Nor will He keep His anger forever. *He has not dealt with us according to our sins, Nor rewarded us according to our iniquities. For as high as the heavens are above the earth, So great is His loving kindness toward those who fear Him. As far as the east is from the west, so far has He removed our transgressions from us.* Just as the father has compassion on his children, *So the Lord has compassion on those who fear Him. For He Himself knows our frame; He is mindful that we are but dust.* As for man, his days are like grass; As a flower of the field, so he flourishes. But the *loving kindness of the Lord is from everlasting to everlasting on those who fear Him, And His righteousness to children's children, To those who keep His covenant and remember His precepts to do them.* The Lord has established His throne in the heavens, *And His sovereignty rules over all.* Bless the Lord, you His angels, Mighty in strength, who performs His word, obeying the voice of His word! Bless the Lord, all you His hosts, you who serve Him, *doing His will.* Bless the Lord, all you works of His, in all places of His dominion; Bless the Lord, O my soul.

Psalm 103:1–15, 17–22

What is the sovereignty of God?

_____

_____

_____

_____

_____

_____

The benefits of knowing Jesus are:

1. He "pardons all of our iniquities."
2. He "heals our diseases."
3. He "redeems our life from the pit."
4. He "crowns us with His loving kindness and compassion."
5. He "satisfies our years with good things."
6. He "renews our spirit."
7. Our " youth is renewed like an eagle."
8. He "performs righteous deeds."

If this is the Lord, why would we not want to sing to Him a new song?

Why would we not praise Him for who He is?

Why would we not want to give Him thanks for what He has done?

Why would we not want to bless His holy name?

Why would we not want to tell of His wonderful works?

Why not?

Sing to the Lord a new song.
Praise God for who He is.
Give Him thanks for what He has done.

> *Bless the Lord, O my soul! O Lord my God, You are very great:* You are *clothed with splendor and majesty,* Covering Yourself with light as with a cloak, Stretching out heaven like a tent curtain. *He established the earth on its foundations,* So that it will not totter forever and ever. You covered it with the deep as with a garment; The waters were standing above the mountains. At Your rebuke they fled, At the sound of Your thunder they hurried away. The mountains rose; and the valleys sank down, To the place which You established for them. You set a boundary that they may not pass over, So that they may not cover the earth. *He sends forth* springs in the valleys; They flow between the mountains; They give drink to every beast of the field; The wild donkeys quench their thirst. Besides them the birds of the heaven dwell; They lift up their voices among the branches. He waters the mountains from His upper chambers; *The earth is satisfied with the fruit of His works. He causes* the grass to grow for the cattle, And the vegetation for the labor of man, so that he may bring forth food from the earth, And wine which makes man's heart glad, So that he may make his face glisten with oil. *And food which sustains man's heart.* The trees of the Lord drink their fill, The cedars of Lebanon which He planted, Where the birds build their nest, And the stork, whose home is in the fir trees. The high mountains are

for the wild goats; The cliffs are a refuge for the SEHHENIM. *He made the moon* for the seasons; *The sun knows* the place of its setting. *You appoint darkness* and it becomes night, In which all the beast of the forest prowl about. The young lions roar after their prey and seek their food from God. When the sun rises they withdrawal and lie down in their dens. Man goes forth to his work and to his labor until evening. *O Lord, how many are Your works! In wisdom You have made them all; The earth is full of Your possessions.* There is the sea great and broad, In which are swarms without number, Animals both small and great. There the ship moves along and Leviathan, which You have formed to support it. They all wait for You to give them their food in due season. You give to them, they gather it up; *You open Your hand , they are satisfied with* good. You hide Your face, they are dismayed; You take away their spirit, they expire and return to dust. *You send forth Your Spirit, they are created, And You renew the face of the ground. Let the glory of the Lord endure forever.* Let the Lord be glad in His works; He looks at the earth and it trembles; He touches the mountains, and they smoke. I will sing to the Lord as long as I live; I will sing praises to my God while I have my being. Let my meditation be pleasing to Him; As for me, I shall be glad in the Lord. Let sinners be consumed from the earth And let the wicked be no more. Bless the Lord O my soul. Praise the Lord.

Psalm 104:1–2, 5–35

In this psalm God describes Himself as clothed with splendor and majesty. He is explaining His wonderful works:

1. He "covers Himself with light."
2. He "stretches out and covers the earth like a tent."
3. He "makes beams is upper chambers."
4. He "makes the clouds His chariot."
5. He "walks upon the wings of the wind."
6. He "established the earth on its foundation."
7. He "gave water to drink."
8. He "gave food to eat."
9. He "sends forth His Spirit and gives life."
10. He "opens His hand."

If God has done all of this, would we not want to sing to Him a new song? If God has done all these things, how much do you think He cares for us? Would we not want to praise Him for who He is? Would we not want to give Him thanks for what He has done?
Sing to the Lord a new song.
Praise God for who He is.
Give Him thanks for what He has done.

> *Praise the Lord! Oh give thanks to the Lord, for He is good;* For His loving kindness is everlasting. Who can speak of the mighty deeds of the Lord, Or who can show forth all His praise? *How blessed are those who keep justice, Who practice righteousness at all times!* Remember me, O Lord, in your favor toward Your people; *visit me with Your salvation,* That I may see the prosperity of Your chosen ones, That I may rejoice in the gladness of Your nation, That I may glory with Your inheri-

tance. We have sinned like our fathers, We have committed iniquity, we have behaved wickedly. Our fathers in Egypt did not understand Your wonders; they did not remember Your abundant kindness, But rebelled by the sea, at the Red Sea. Nevertheless *He saved them for the sake of His name, that He might make His power known.* Thus He rebuked the Red Sea and it dried up, And He led them through the deeps, as through the wilderness. So He saved them from the hand of the one who hated them, And remembered them from the land of the enemy. The waters covered their adversaries; Not one of them was left. *Then they believed His words; they sang His praise.*

Psalm 106:1–12

God saved us for His name's sake to make His power known. We are ambassadors for Jesus. He has redeemed us that we might display His glory. When God redeems us, we are in a transforming process to practice righteousness. In this process He gives us a new song to sing in praising Him for who He is and giving Him thanks for what He has done.

Sing to the Lord a new song.
Praise God for who He is.
Give Him thanks for what He Has done.

> *Oh give thanks to the Lord, for He is good, For His loving kindness is everlasting. Let the redeemed of the Lord say so, Whom He has redeemed from the hand of the adversary* And gathered from the lands, From the east and from the west, From the north and from the south; Their soul fainted within them.

Then they cried out to the Lord in their trouble; He delivered them out of their distress. He led them also by a straight way, to go to an inhabited city. Let them give thanks to the Lord for His loving kindness, And for His wonders to the sons of men! For He has satisfied their thirsty soul, And the hungry soul He has filled with what is good. Therefore He humbled their heart with labor; They stumbled and there was none to help. Then they cried out to the Lord in their trouble; *He Saved them* out of their distresses. He brought them out of darkness and the shadow of death And broke their bands apart. Let them *give thanks* to the Lord *for His loving kindness,* And *for His wonders* to the sons of men! *Then they cried out to the Lord in their trouble; He saved them out of their distress. He sent His word and healed them, And delivered them from their destructions. Let them give thanks to the Lord for His loving kindness, And His wonders to the sons of men! Let them also offer sacrifices of thanksgiving, And tell of His works with joyful singing.* Those who go down to the sea in ships, Who do business on great waters; They have seen the works of the Lord and His wonders in the deep. For *He spoke and raised* up a stormy wind, which lifted up the waves of the sea. They rose up to the heavens, they went down to the depths; Their soul melted away in their misery. They reeled and staggered like a drunken man, And were at their wits' end. Then they cried to the Lord in their trouble, And He *brought them out of their* distress. *He caused* the storm to be still, So that the waves of the sea were hushed. Then they were glad because they were quiet. So *He guided* them out to their desired haven. Let them *give thanks* to the Lord for His loving kindness, and for His wonders to the sons of men! Let them extol Him also in the congregation of the people, And *praise Him* at the seat of the elders. *He changes rivers* into a wilderness and springs of water into a thirsty ground; A fruitful land into a salt waste, because of the wickedness of those who dwell in it. *He changes a wilderness* into a pool of water; And a dry land into springs of water; And there He makes the hungry dwell, So that they may establish an inhabited city, And sow fields and plant vineyards, And gather a fruitful harvest. Also He blesses them and they multiply greatly, And He does not let their cattle decrease. When they are diminished and bowed down Through oppression, misery and sorrow, He pours contempt upon princes And makes them wander in a pathless waste. *But He sets the needy securely on high away from affliction, and makes his families like a flock. The upright see it and are glad; But all unrighteousness shuts its mouth. Who is wise? Let him give heed to these things, And consider the loving kindness of the Lord.*

Psalm 107:1–3, 5–9, 13–43

With all of David's trouble, he has experienced the Lord down deep in the inner being.

The promises of the Lord:

1. The Lord "redeems" us.
2. He "saves" us.
3. He "delivers" us.
4. He "leads" us.
5. He "raises us up."

6. He "guides us."

7. He "changes"—transforms—everything. If God can transform my life, he will be able to transform your life too. It's your choice.

List all the works of God in this psalm.

_____

_____

_____

_____

_____

_____

As God did these things for David, He desires to do for us. When we experience Jesus as David did, in our inner most being, we can extol His name, sing a new song to Him, praise His name for who He is, and give Him thanks for what He has done.

Sing to the Lord a new song.
Praise God for who He is.
Give Him thanks for what He has done.

> *Praise the Lord! I will give thanks to the Lord with all my heart, In the company of the upright and in the assembly. Great are the works of the Lord; They are studied by all who delight in them. Splendid and*

majestic is His work. And His righteousness endures forever. He has made His wonders to be remembered; The Lord is gracious and compassionate. He has given food to those who fear Him; He will remember His covenant forever. He has made known to His people the power of His works, In giving them the heritage of the nations. The works of His hands are truth and justice; all His precepts are sure. They are upheld forever and ever; They are performed in truth and uprightness. *He has* sent redemption to His people; *He has* ordained His covenant forever; Holy and awesome is His name. The fear of the Lord is the beginning of wisdom; a good understanding have all those who do His commandments; His praise endures forever.

Psalm 111

When we see God in all His splendor, majesty, righteousness, power, and holiness, we will want to keep His commandments. We will want to sing to Him a new song and praise Him for His awesomeness toward us.

What are the promises in this psalm?

_____

_____

_____

_____

_____

Sing to the Lord a new song.
Praise God for who He is.
Give Him thanks for what He has done.

> *Praise the Lord! How blessed is the man who fears the Lord. Who greatly delights in His commandments.* His descendants will be mighty on the earth; *The generation of the upright will be blessed.* Wealth and riches are in His house, And His righteousness endures forever. *Light arises in the darkness for the upright; He is gracious, and compassionate,* and *righteous. For he will never be shaken;* The righteous will be redeemed forever. He will not fear evil tidings; *his heart is steadfast, trusting in the Lord. his heart is upheld, he will not fear,* Until he looks with satisfaction on his adversaries. He has given freely to the poor, His righteousness endures forever; His horn will be exalted in honor.
>
> Psalm 112:1–4, 6–9

If we fear the Lord, and delight ourselves in His commandments, we will be blessed, because "His righteousness endures forever." Our heart will be steadfast, and "we will never be shaken." Then we will be able to sing a new song to the Lord, praise Him for who He is, and give Him thanks for what He has done.

Sing to the Lord a new song.
Praise God for who He is.
Give Him thanks for what He has done.

> *Praise the Lord! Praise, O servants of the Lord, Praise the name of the Lord. Blessed be the name of the Lord,* From this time forth and forever. From the ris-

ing of the sun to its setting *The name of the Lord is to be praised. The Lord is high above nations; His glory is above the heavens.* Who is like the Lord our God, Who is enthroned on high, Who humbles Himself to behold the things that are in heaven and on the earth? He raises the poor from the dust and lifts the needy from the ash heap.

Psalm 113:1–7

How is God described in this psalm?

Here God invites us to fall on our knees and cry to Him for help. He is certainly willing and more than able to help us in times of need. He will lift us up and put us on firm ground. Once we have experienced the glory of the Lord, we are able to sing to Him a new song. We are able to praise Him for who He is and give Him thanks for what He has done for us.

_____

_____

_____

_____

Sing to the Lord a new song.
Praise God for who He is.
Give Him thanks for what He has done.

I love the Lord, because He hears my voice and my supplications. Because He has inclined His ear to me, therefore I shall call upon Him as long as I live. The cords of death encompassed me and the terrors of SHEOL Came upon me: I found distress and sorrow. Then I called upon the name of the Lord: "O Lord, I beseech You, save my life!" Gracious is the Lord, and righteous: Yes, our God is compassionate. The Lord preserves the simple; I was brought low, and He saved me. Return to your rest, O my soul, For the Lord has dealt bountifully with you. For You have rescued my soul from death, my eyes from tears, My feet from stumbling. I shall walk before the Lord in the land of the living. I believed when I said, "I am greatly afflicted." I shall lift up the cup of salvation And call upon the name of the Lord. I shall pay my vows to the Lord, Oh may it be in the presence of all His people. Precious in the sight of the Lord is the death His godly ones. O Lord, surely I am Your servant, I am Your servant, the son of Your handmaid, You have loosed my bonds. To You I shall offer a sacrifice of *thanksgiving,* And *call upon the name of the Lord.* I shall pay my vows to the Lord, Oh may it be in the presence of all His people, In the courts of the Lord's house, In the midst of You, O Jerusalem. Praise the Lord.

Psalm 116:1–10, 13–19

Make your list of characteristics that define the name of the Lord.

_____

_____

_____

Sing to the Lord a new song.
Praise God for who He is.
Give Him thanks for what He has done.

Give thanks to the Lord for He is good; For His loving kindness is everlasting. *Oh let those who fear the Lord say, "His loving kindness is everlasting." From my distress I called upon the Lord; The Lord answered me and set me in a large place. The Lord is for me; I will not fear. What can man do to me? The Lord is for me among those who help me. Therefore I will look with satisfaction on those who hate me. It is better to take refuge in the Lord than to trust in man.* It is better to take refuge in the Lord than to trust in princes. You pushed me violently so that I was falling, *But the Lord helped me. The Lord is my strength and my song, And He has become my salvation.* The sound *of joyful shouting and salvation is in the tents of the righteous; the right hand of the Lord does valiantly. The right hand of the Lord is exalted; I will not die, but live, And tell of the works of the Lord.* The Lord has disciplined me severely, but He has not given me over to death. Open to me the gates of righteousness; I shall enter through them, *I shall give thanks to the Lord.* This is the gate of the Lord; The righteous will enter through it. *I shall give thanks to You, for You have answered me, And You have become my salvation.* The stone which the builders rejected Has become the chief corner stone. This is the Lord's doing; It is marvelous in our eyes. This is the day which the Lord has made; let us rejoice and be glad in it. Oh Lord, do save, we beseech you, do send prosperity! Blessed is the one who comes in the name of the Lord. We have blessed you from the house of the Lord. The Lord is God, and He has given us light; Bind the festival sacrifice with cords to the horns of the altar. *You are my God and I will give thanks to You; You are my God, I extol You. Give thanks to the Lord for He is good; For His loving kindness is everlasting.*

Psalm 118:1, 3–9, 13–29

When we fall on our knees in the times of stress and trouble, God will hear us and answer us. God is for us and wants to help us. The Lord will deliver us and set us in a large place. When He does that, we are able to sing to Him a new song. We can praise Him for who He is and give Him thanks for what He has done.

What are the promises from this psalm?

_____

_____

_____

_____

_____

Sing to the Lord a new song.
Praise God for who He is.
Give Him thanks for what He has done.

I will lift up my eyes to the mountains From where shall my help come? My help comes from the Lord,

Who made heaven and earth. *He will not allow your foot to slip;* He who keeps you will not slumber. *The Lord is your keeper; The Lord is your* shade on you right hand. The sun will not smite you by day Nor the moon by night, *The Lord will protect you from all evil; He will keep your soul. The Lord will guard your going out and your coming in from this time forth* and forever.

Psalm 121:1–3, 5–8

When we look to the Lord, He will be our help. He will protect us and guard us from evil. He watches over our comings and our goings. When we experience the protection of the Lord, we will be able to sing to Him a new song. With confidence we can praise Him for who He is and give Him thanks for what He has done. Characteristics of the Lord from this psalm:

1. Helper
2. Maker
3. Lifter
4. Keeper
5. Shade
6. Protector
7. Guard
8. Strength

Sing to the lord a new song.
Praise God for who He is.
Give Him thanks for what He has done.

I will give thanks with all my heart; I will sing praises to You before the gods. I will bow down toward Your holy temple And give thanks to Your name for Your loving kindness and Your truth; for You have magnified Your word according to *all Your name.* On the day I called, You answered me; You made me bold with strength in my soul. All the kings of the earth will give thanks to You, Oh Lord, when they have heard the words of Your mouth. And they will sing of the ways of the Lord, for great is the glory of the Lord. For though the Lord is exalted, yet He regards the lowly, but the haughty He knows from afar. Though I walk in the midst of trouble, *You will revive me;* You will stretch forth Your hand against the wrath of my enemies, And Your right hand will save me. The Lord will accomplish what concerns me; Your loving kindness, O Lord, is everlasting; do not forsake the works of Your hands.

Psalm 138

Consider all the characteristics of the Lord when the Bible states "all your name."
What are the promises from this psalm?

What does the glory of the Lord look like to you?

_____

_____

_____

_____

_____

Sing to the Lord a new song.
Praise God for who He is.
Give Him thanks for what He has done.

> Blessed be the Lord; my *rock*, Who *trains* my hands for war, And my fingers for battle; My *loving kindness and my fortress,*
>
> *My stronghold and my deliverer, My shield and He in whom I take refuge, Who subdues* my people under me. O Lord, what is man, that you take knowledge of him? Or the son of man that you think of him? Man is like a mere breath; His days are like a passing shadow. *I will sing a new song to You,* O God; Upon a harp of ten strings *I will sing praise to You,* Who gives *salvation* to kings, *Who rescued David* His servant from the evil sword. *Rescue and deliver me* out of the hand of the aliens, Whose mouth speak deceit And whose right hand is a right hand of falsehood. Let our sons in their youth be as *grown-up Plants,* And our daughters as *corner pillars* fashioned as for a palace; Let our garners be full, furnishing every kind of produce, And our flocks bring forth thousands and ten thousands in our fields; *How blessed are the people who are so situated; How blessed are the people whose God is Lord!*

Psalm 144:1–4, 9–13, 15

List at least twenty characteristics of God in this psalm.

What does the word *blessed* mean to you?

What are the promises of the Lord?

_____

_____

_____

_____

_____

_____

_____

_____

What does it mean to be "so situated?"

_____

_____

_____

_____

Sing to the Lord a new song.
Praise God for who He is.
Give Him thanks for what He has done.

I will extol you, my God, O King, and *I will bless Your name forever* and ever. Every day I will bless You, And I will praise Your name forever and ever. *Great is the Lord and highly* to be praised, and *His greatness is unsearchable.* One generation *will praise Your works to another,* and shall *declare Your mighty acts. On the glorious splendor of Your majesty And on Your wonderful works, I will meditate.* Men *shall speak of the power* of Your *awesome acts, And I will tell of Your greatness.* They shall *eagerly utter* the memory of Your abundant goodness and will *shout joyfully* of Your righteousness. *The Lord is gracious and merciful;* slow to anger and great in loving kindness. The Lord is good to all, and His mercies are over all His works. All Your works shall give thanks to You O Lord, And Your godly ones shall bless You. They *shall speak of the glory* of Your Kingdom and *talk of Your power;* to make known to the sons of men Your mighty acts and the glory of the majesty of Your Kingdom, Your Kingdom is an everlasting Kingdom, And Your dominion endures throughout all generations. The *Lord sustains all* who fall And *raises up* all who are bowed down. The eyes of all look to You, *And You give them their food in due time.* You open up Your hand And *satisfy the desire* of every living thing. *The Lord is righteous in all His ways and kind in all His deeds.* The *Lord is near* to all who call upon Him, to all who call upon Him in truth. He will *fulfill the desires* of those who fear Him; *He will also hear* their cry and will *save them.* The *Lord keeps* all who love Him, but all the wicked He will destroy. My mouth will speak the praise of the Lord, and all flesh will bless His holy name forever and ever.

Psalm 145

When we have experienced the fullness of God; all His glory, power, grace, mercy, forgiveness, and His presence, we cannot keep it to ourselves. We will want to extol Him, praise Him, and give Him thanks.

Sing to the Lord a new song.
Praise God for who He is.
Give Him thanks for what He has done.

> Praise the Lord! Praise the Lord O my soul! *I will praise the Lord while I live; I will sing praises to my God while I have my being.* Do not trust in princes, In mortal man, in whom there is no salvation. His spirit departs, he returns to the earth; In that very day his thoughts perish. *How blessed is he* whose help is the God of Jacob, Whose *hope is in the Lord his God,* Who made heaven and earth, The sea and all that is in them; Who keeps faith forever; Who *executes justice* for the oppressed; Who gives food to the hungry. *The Lord sets the prisoners free.* The *Lord opens* the eyes of the blind; The *Lord raises up* those who are bowed down; The Lord loves the righteous. *The Lord protects* the strangers; He supports the fatherless and the widow, *The Lord will reign forever,* Your God, O Zion, to all generations. Praise the Lord.
>
> Psalm 146

What are the promises in this psalm?

Why do and why will you sing praise to God?

How are you able to sing praise to God?

_____

_____

_____

_____

_____

_____

_____

_____

_____

List more than twelve characteristics of God from this psalm.

Sing to the Lord a new song.
Praise God for who He is.
Give Him thanks for what He has done.

> Praise the Lord! For *it is good to sing praises to our God;* For *it is pleasant and praise is becoming. He heals the brokenhearted and binds up* their wounds. *He counts* the number of stars; *He gives* names to all of them. Great is our Lord and *abundant in*

strength; His *understanding is infinite.* The Lord *supports* the afflicted; He *brings down* the wicked to the ground. *Sing to the Lord with thanksgiving. Sing praises to our God* on the lyre, Who *covers the heavens* with clouds. Who *provides rain* for the earth, Who *makes grass to grow* on the mountains. He gives to the beast its food, And to the young ravens which cry. He does not delight in the strength of the horse; He does not take pleasure in the legs of man. *The Lord favors those who fear Him, Those who wait for His loving kindness.* Praise the Lord O Jerusalem! Praise your God, O Zion! For He has strengthened the bars of your gates; He has blessed your sons within you. He makes peace in your borders; *He satisfies you* with the finest of wheat. He sends forth His command to the earth; His word runs very swiftly. *He gives* snow like wool; He scatters the frost like ashes. He casts forth His ice as fragments; Who can stand before His cold? *He sends forth* His word and melts them; *He causes* His wind to blow and the waters to flow. *He declares* His word to Jacob, His statutes and His ordinances to Israel. He has not dealt thus with any nation; And as for His ordinances, they have not known them.
Praise the Lord!

Psalm 147:1, 3–20

List all the characteristics of the Lord in this psalm.

List the wonderful deeds of the Lord.

_____

_____

_____

_____

_____

_____

_____

_____

Why is it good to sing praise to God?

What kind of effect does singing a new song to the Lord have on our being?

_____

_____

_____

_____

_____

_____

Sing to the Lord a new song.
Praise God for who He is.
Give Him thanks for what He has done.

> Praise the Lord! Praise the Lord from the heavens; Praise Him in the heights! Praise Him all the stars and light, Praise Him highest heavens, *Both young men and virgins; Old men and children. Let them Praise the name of the Lord, For His name alone is exalted; His glory is above the earth and heaven. And He has lifted up a horn for His people. Praise for all His godly ones!* Even for the sons of Israel, A people near Him. Praise the Lord!
>
> Psalm 148:1–4, 12–14

The word *praise* is listed eight times in this verse.

Study how many times the word *praise* is used in the entire Bible.

_____

_____

_____

_____

_____

_____

_____

Sing to the Lord a new song.
Praise God for who He is.
Give Him thanks for what He has done.

> Praise the Lord! *Sing to the Lord a new song,* And His praise in the congregation of the godly ones. Let Israel be glad in his maker; Let the sons of Zion rejoice in their King. Let them praise His name with dancing; Let them sing praise to Him with TIMBREL and lyre. *For the Lord takes pleasure in His people; He will beautify the afflicted with salvation. Let the godly ones exalt in glory;* Let them Sing for joy on their beds. Let the high praises of God be in their mouth And *the two-edged sword in their* hand, To execute vengeance on the nations And punishment on the peoples, To bind their kings with chains and their nobles with fetters of iron, To execute on them the judgment written, This is an honor for all His godly ones. Praise the Lord!
>
> Psalm 149

According to this psalm, we are to "sing to the Lord a new song," a song of praise. Allow God to transform you life, and He will work wonderful things in your life.

Not only in these verses, but throughout psalms, the Lord takes pleasure in us and also delights in us. If He does these things, will He not take care of us?

_____

_____

_____

_____

Sing to the Lord a new song.
Praise God for who He is.
Give Him thanks for what He has done.

> Praise the Lord! Praise God in His sanctuary;
> Praise Him in His mighty expanse. Praise Him
> for His mighty deeds; Praise Him according to
> His excellent greatness. Praise Him with trum-
> pet sound, Praise Him with harp and lyre. Praise
> Him with TIMBREL and dancing; Praise Him
> with stringed instruments and pipe, Praise Him
> with loud cymbals; Praise Him with resounding
> cymbals, let everything that has breath, Praise the
> Lord.
>
> Psalm 150

The command is to "Praise God!" So, to be able to "sing
a new song to the Lord," what are you going to do?

Sing to the Lord a new song.
Praise God for who He is.
Give Him thanks for what He Has done.

> *Sing to the Lord a new song!*
> Play skillfully with a shout of joy.
>
> Psalm 33:3

He put a new song in my mouth,
A song of praise to our God.

Psalm 40:3

Sing to the Lord a new song!
Sing to the Lord, all the earth.

Psalm 96:1

O sing to the Lord a new song!
For He has done wonderful things,
His right hand and His holy arm has gained the
victory for Him.

Psalm 98:1

I will sing a new song to You, O Lord;
Upon a harp of ten strings I will sing praises to
You.

Psalm 144:9

Sing to the Lord a new song
Sing praise from the end of the earth.

Isaiah 42:10

What is the main idea in the verses you just read?

_____

_____

_____

The main topic of the following verses is singing praise to God. There are over thirty verses that say "sing praise" to God. Search the Bible, using your concordance, and find all the verses that talk about singing and/or praising God.

_____

_____

_____

_____

_____

Then Moses and the sons of Israel sang this song to the Lord and said, I will sing to the Lord for He is highly exulted;
    The Lord is my strength and my song, and He has become my salvation;
    This is my God, and I will praise Him;
    My father's God, and I will extol Him.
    The Lord is a warrior;
    The Lord is His name.

Exodus 15:1–3

Hear, O kings; give ear, O rulers!
I will sing, I will sing praise to the Lord, the God of Israel.

Judges 5:3

I will give thanks to the Lord according to His righteousness and will sing praise to the name of the Most High.

Psalm 7:17

I will be glad and exult in You;
I will sing praises to Your name, O Most High.

Psalm 9:2

Sing praises to the Lord, who dwells in ZION;
Declare among the peoples His deeds.

Psalm 9:11

I will sing to the Lord,
Because He has dwelt bountifully with me.

Psalm 13:6

Therefore I will give thanks to You among the nations, O Lord, and I will sing praises to Your name.

Psalm 18:49

And now my head will be lifted up above my enemies around me, and I will offer in His tent sacrifices with shouts of joy; I will sing, yes, I will sing praises to the Lord.

Psalm 27:6

That my soul may sing praises to You and not be silent. O my Lord, I will give thanks to You forever.

Psalm 30:12

Sing praises to God, sing praises; sing praises to our King, sing praises. For God is King over all the earth; sing praises with a skillful psalm.

Psalm 47:6–7

My heart is steadfast, O God, my heart is steadfast; I will sing, yes I will sing praises to Your name!

Psalm 57:7

O my strength, I will sing praises to You; For God is my stronghold, the God who shows me loving kindness.

Psalm 59:17

Sing to God, O kingdoms of the earth, sing praises To the Lord.

Psalm 68:32

I will sing of the loving kindness of the Lord forever; to all generations I will make known Your faithfulness with my mouth.

Psalm 89:1

It is good to give thanks to the Lord and sing praises to Your name, O Most High.

Psalm 92:1

Sing praise to the Lord in song, for He has done excellent things; let this be known throughout the earth.
Sing to the Lord a new song!
Praise the Lord for who He is!

Isaiah 12:5

_____

_____

_____

Write down your thoughts, in your own words, who
God is.

_____

_____

_____

_____

There are over twenty-five verses in the Bible that say,
"Give thanks to the Lord."

Find them and write them down.

_____

_____

_____

> Therefore I will give thanks to You, O Lord,
> among the nations, And I will sing praise to Your
> name.
>
> 2 Samuel 22:50

Oh give thanks to the Lord, call upon His name;
make known His deeds among the peoples.

1 Chronicles 16:8

O give thanks to the Lord, for He is good; for His
loving kindness is everlasting.
Then say, "Save us, O God of our salvation,"
And gather us and deliver us from the nations,
to give thanks to Your holy name, and to glory in
Your praise."

1 Chronicles 16:34–35

Therefore I will give thanks to You among the
nations, O Lord, and I will sing praise to Your
name.

Psalm 18:49

Sing praise to the Lord, You His godly ones. Give
thanks to His holy name.

Psalm 30:4

That my soul may sing praises to You and not be
silent. O my God, I will give thanks to You forever.

Psalm 30:12

I will give thanks in the great congregation;
I will praise You among the mighty throng.

Psalm 35:18

We give thanks to You, O Lord, we give thanks.
Men declare Your wondrous works.

Psalm 75:1

So we Your people and the sheep of Your pasture will give thanks to You forever. To all generations we will tell of Your praise.

Psalm 79:13

Oh give thanks to the Lord, call upon His name; make known His deeds among the peoples, Sing to Him, sing praises to Him;
Speak of all His wonders.

Psalm 105:1–2

Praise the Lord!
Oh give thanks to the Lord, for He is good;
His loving kindness is everlasting.

Psalm 106:1

Oh give thanks to the Lord for He is good, for His loving kindness is everlasting. Let the redeemed of the Lord say so, Whom He has redeemed us from the adversary.

Psalm 107:1-2

Praise the Lord!
I will give thanks to the Lord with all my heart.
In the company of the upright and in the assembly.

Psalm 111:1

In your own words, what do the above verses say to you?

_____

_____

_____

In your Bible search for other verses that talk about giving thanks.

_____

_____

_____

What has God done for you personally, nationally, around the world, spiritually, physically, mentally, emotionally?

_____

_____

_____

_____

_____

Sing to the Lord a new song.
Praise the Lord for who He is.
Give Him thanks for what He has done.

In the beginning was the Word, and the Word was with God, and the Word was God. He was in the beginning with God. All things came into being through Him, and apart from Him nothing came into being that has come into being. In Him was life, and the life was the Light of men. The Light shines in the darkness, and the darkness did not comprehend it. Then came a man sent by God, whose name was John. He came as a witness, to testify about the Light, so that *all might believe through Him.* He was not the Light, but came to testify about the Light. *There was the true Light which, coming into the world, enlightens every man.* He was in the world, and the world was made through Him, and the world did not know Him. He came to His own, and those who were His own did not receive Him. *But as many as received Him, to them He gave the right to become children of God, even those who believe in His name, who were born not of blood, nor of the will of the flesh nor of the will of man, but of God.* And the Word became flesh, and dwelt among us, and *we saw His glory,* glory as of the only one from the Father, *full of grace and truth.* John testified about Him and cried out, saying, "this was He of whom I said, He who comes after me has a higher rank than I, for He existed before me." *For of His fullness we have all received grace upon grace. For the Law was given through Moses; grace and truth were realized through Jesus Christ.*

John 1:1–17

List six characteristics of the nature of Christ.

_____

_____

_____

From this portion of John 1, Jesus is the "Light of the world."

What does "light" and "dark" refer to here?

_____

_____

_____

_____

Sing to the Lord a new song.
Praise God for who He is.
Give Him thanks for what He has done.

> Now there was a man of the Pharisees, named Nicodemus, a ruler of the Jews; this man came to Jesus by night and said to Him, "Rabbi, we know that You have come from God as a teacher; for no one can do these signs that You do unless God is with Him." *Jesus answered and said to him, "Truly, truly, I say to you, unless one is born again he cannot see the* Kingdom of God." Nicodemus said to Him, "How can a man be born when he is old?" He cannot enter a second time into his mother's womb and be born, can he?" *Jesus answered, "Truly, truly,*

I say to you, unless one is born of water and the Spirit he cannot enter into the Kingdom of God. That which is born of the flesh is flesh, and that which is born of the Spirit is spirit. Do not be amazed that I said to you, "you must be born again." The wind blows where it wishes and you hear the sound of it, but do not know where it comes from and where it is going; So is everyone who is born of the Spirit." Nicodemus said to him, "How can this be?"

Jesus answered and said to him, "Are you the teacher of Israel and do not understand these things? "Truly, truly, I say to you, we speak of what we know and testify of what we have seen, and you do not accept our testimony. If I told you earthly things and you do not believe, *how will you believe if I tell you heavenly things?* No one has ascended into heaven, but He who descended from heaven; the Son of Man. As Moses lifted up the serpent in the wilderness, even so must the Son of man be lifted up; so that *whoever believes in Him might have eternal life. For God so loved the world, that He gave His only begotten Son, that whoever believes in Him shall not perish, but have eternal life. For God did not send His Son into the world to judge the world, But that the world might be saved trough Him. He who believes* in Him is not judged; he who does not believe is judged already because he has not believed in the name of the only begotten Son of God. This is the judgment, that the Light has come into the world, and men loved the darkness rather than the Light, for their deeds were evil. For everyone who does evil hates the Light, and does not come to the Light for fear that his deeds will be exposed, *but he who practices the truth comes to the Light, so that his deeds may be manifested as having been wrought in God."*

In your own words, what does this portion of Scripture say?

_____

_____

_____

_____

What does it mean to be "born of the Spirit?"

_____

_____

_____

What does "wrought in God" mean?

_____

_____

_____

Sing to the Lord a new song.
Praise God for who He is.
Give Him thanks for what He has done.

> *Therefore Jesus answered and was saying to them, "Truly, truly, I say to you, the Son can do nothing*

of Himself, unless it is something He sees the Father doing; for whatever the Father does, these things the Son also does in like manner. For the Father loves the Son, and shows Him all things that He Himself is doing; and the Father will show Him greater works than these, so that you may marvel. For just as the Father raises the dead and gives them life, even so the Son gives life to who He wishes. For not even the Father judges anyone, but He has given all judgment to the Son, so that all will *honor the Son* even as they honor the Father. He who does not honor the Son does not honor the Father who sent Him. *"Truly, truly, I say to you, he who hears My word, and believes Him who sent Me, has eternal life,* and does not come into judgment, *but has passed out of death into life. "Truly, truly, I say to you, an hour is coming and now is, when the dead will hear the voice of the Son of God, and those who hear will live.* For just as the Father has life in Himself, even so He gave to the Son also to have life in Himself; and He gave Him authority to execute judgment, because He is the Son of Man. Do not marvel at this; for an hour is coming, in which all who are in the tombs will hear His voice, and will come forth; *those who did the good deeds to a resurrection of life,* those who committed the evil deeds to a resurrection of judgment. I can do nothing on My own initiative. As I hear, I judge; and My judgment is just, because I do not seek My own will, but the will of Him who sent me."

John 5:19–30

In your own words, how can we see what the Father is doing?

_____

_____

_____

Who gives life?

_____

_____

_____

What kind of life?

_____

_____

_____

How can we experience life?

_____

_____

_____

Sing to the Lord a new song.
Praise God for who He is.
Give Him thanks for what He has done.

Jesus answered them and said, "Truly, truly, I say to you, You seek Me, not because you saw signs, but because you ate of the loaves and were filled. Do not work for food which perishes, but for the food which endures to eternal life, which the Son of Man will give you, For on Him the Father, God, *has set His seal."* Therefore they said to Him, "What shall we do, so that we may work the works of God?" Jesus answered and said to them, *"This is the work of God, that you believe in Him who He has sent."* So they said to Him, "What then do You do for a sign, so that we may see, and believe You? What work do You perform? Our fathers ate the manna in the wilderness; as it is written, He gave them bread out of heaven to eat." Jesus then said to them, *"Truly, truly, I say to you, it is not Moses who has given you the bread out of heaven, but it is My Father who gives you true bread out of heaven. For the bread of God is that which comes down out of heaven, and gives life to the world."* Then they said to Him, "Lord, always give us this bread." Jesus said to them, *"I am the bread of life; he who comes to Me will not hunger, and he who believes in Me will never thirst.* But I said to you that you have seen Me, and yet do not believe. All that the Father gives Me will come to Me, and the one that comes to Me I will certainly not cast out. For I have come down from heaven, not to do My own will, but the will of Him who sent Me. This is the will of Him who sent Me, that of all He has given Me I lose nothing. For this is the will of My *Father, that everyone who beholds the Son and believes in Him has eternal life, and I myself will raise Him up on the last day.*" Therefore the Jews were grumbling about Him, because He said, "I am the bread that came down out of heaven." They were saying, "Is this not Jesus, the son of Joseph, whose father and mother we know? How does He now say, 'I have come down out of heaven?'" Jesus answered and said to them, "Do not grumble amongst yourselves. No one can come to Me unless the Father who sent Me draws him; and I will raise him up on the last day. It is written in the prophets, and they all shall be *taught of God.* Everyone who has heard and learned from the Father, comes to Me. Not that anyone has seen the Father, except the one who is from God; He has seen the Father. *Truly, truly, I say to you, he who believes has eternal life. I am the bread of life.* Your fathers ate the manna in the wilderness, and they died. *This is the bread which comes down from heaven, so that you may eat of it and not die. I am the living bread that came down from heaven; if anyone eats of this bread, he will live forever; and the bread also which I give for the life of the world is My flesh.*" Then the Jews began to argue with one another, saying, "How can this man give us His flesh to eat?" So Jesus said to them, "Truly, truly, I say to you, unless you eat the flesh of the Son of Man and drink His blood, you have no life in yourselves. He who eats My flesh and drinks My blood has eternal life, And I will raise him up on the last day. For My flesh is true food and My blood is true drink. He who eats My flesh and drinks My blood abides in Me and I in him. As the living Father sent Me, and I live because of the Father so he who eats Me, he also will live because of Me. This is the bread which

came down out of heaven; not as the fathers ate
and died; *He who eats this bread will live forever.*"

John 6:26–58

Who is the true bread of life?

_____

_____

_____

Who gives eternal life?

_____

_____

_____

Who is God?

_____

_____

_____

Who is Jesus?

_____

_____

_____

_____

How can we live forever?

_____

_____

_____

Sing to the Lord a new song.
Praise God for who He is.
Give Him thanks for what He has done.

> *Then Jesus again spoke to them, saying, "I am the Light of the world; He who follows me will not walk in darkness, but will have the Light of life."* So the Pharisees said to Him, "You are testifying about Yourself; Your testimony is not true." Jesus answered and said to them, "Even if I testify about Myself, *My testimony is true,* for I know where I came from and where I am going; You judge according to the flesh; I am not judging anyone. But even if I do judge, *My judgment is true;* for I am not alone in it, but I and the Father who sent Me. Even in your law it has been written that the testimony of two men is true. I am He who testifies about Myself, and the Father who sent Me testifies about Me." So they were saying to Him, "Where is the Father?" Jesus answered, "You know neither Me nor My Father; *if you knew Me, you would know My Father also."* These words He

spoke in the treasury, as He taught in the temple; And no one seized Him because His hour had not come. Then He said again to them, "I go away, and you will seek Me, and will die in your sins; where I am going, you cannot come." So the Jews were saying, "Surely He will not kill Himself, will He, since He says, *'Where I am going you cannot come'?" And He was saying to them, "You are from below, I am from above; you are of this world, I am not of this world. Therefore I said to you that you will die in your sins; for unless you believe that I am He, you will die in your sins."* So they were saying to Him, "Who are You?" Jesus said to them "What have I been saying to you from the beginning? I have many things to speak and to judge concerning you, but He who sent Me is true; and the things I heard from Him, these things I speak to the world." They did not realize that He had been speaking to them about the Father. So Jesus said, "When you lift up the Son of Man, then you will know that I am He, and I do nothing on My own initiative, but I speak these things as the Father taught Me. And He who sent Me is with Me*; He has not left Me alone, for I always do the things that are pleasing to Him." As He spoke these things, many came to believe in Him.* So Jesus was saying to those Jews who had believed Him, *"If you continue in My Word, then you truly are disciples of Mine; And you will know the truth and the truth will make you free.* They answered Him, "We are Abrahams descendants and have never yet been enslaved to anyone; how is it that You say we will become free?" *Jesus answered them, "Truly, truly I say to you, everyone who commits sin is the slave to sin. Jesus said to them, "If God were your Father, you would love Me,* for I proceeded forth and have come from God, for I have not even come on My own initiative, but He sent Me. Why do you not understand what I am saying? It is because you cannot hear My Word. You are of your father, the devil, and you want to do the desires of your father. He was a murderer from the beginning, and does not stand in the truth because there is no truth in him. When ever he speaks a lie, he speaks from his own nature, for he is a liar and the father of lies. But because I speak the truth, you do not believe Me. Which one of you convicts Me of sin? He who is of God hears the Words of God; for this reason you do not hear them, because you are not of God." The Jews answered and said to Him, "Do we not say rightly that You are a Samaritan and have a demon?" Jesus answered, "I do not have a demon; but I honor My Father, and you dishonor Me. But I do not seek My glory; there is one who seeks and judges. *Truly, truly, I say to you, if any one keeps My Word he will never see death.*" The Jews said to Him, "Now we know You have a demon. Abraham died, and the prophets also; and You say, 'If anyone keeps My word, he will never taste death.'" Surely You are not greater than our father Abraham, who died? the prophets died too; who do You make Yourself out to be?" Jesus answered, "If I glorify Myself, My glory is nothing; it is My Father who glorifies Me, of whom you say, 'He is our God'; and you have not come to know Him, but I know Him; and if I say I do not know Him, I will be a liar like you, but I do know Him and keep His Word. Your father Abraham rejoiced to see My day, and he saw it and was glad." So the Jews said to Him, "You are not yet fifty years old, and You have seen Abraham?" Jesus said to them, "Truly, truly, I say to you, before Abraham was born, I am."

John 8:12–34, 42–55

In your own words, list all the characteristics of who Jesus is.

_____

_____

_____

What are the things that are pleasing to God?

_____

_____

_____

How do you hear the words of God?

_____

_____

Sing to the Lord a new song.
Praise God for who He is.
Give Him thanks for what He has done.

"Truly, truly. I say to you, he who does not enter by

the door into the fold of the sheep, but climbs up some other way, he is a thief and a robber. But he who enters by the door is a shepherd of the sheep. To him the door keeper opens, and the sheep hear his voice, and he calls his own sheep by name and leads them out. When he puts forth all his own, he goes ahead of them, and the sheep follow him because they know his voice. A stranger they simply will not follow, but will flee from him, because they do not know the voice of strangers." This figure of speech Jesus spoke to them, but they did not understand what those things were which He had been saying to them. *So Jesus said to them again, "Truly, truly, I say to you I* am *the door of the sheep.* All who came before Me are thieves and robbers, but the sheep did not hear them. *I am the door; if anyone enters through Me, he will be saved, and will go in and out and find pasture.* The thief only comes to steal, kill and destroy; *I come that they may have life, and have it more abundantly. I am the good shepherd: the good shepherd lays down His life for the sheep.* He who is a hired hand, and not a shepherd, who is not the owner of the sheep, sees the wolf coming, and leaves the sheep and flees, and the wolf snatches them and scatters them. He flees because he is a hired hand and is not concerned about the sheep. *I am the good shepherd, and I know My own and My own know Me. Even as the Father knows Me I know the Father; and I lay down My life for the sheep.* I have other sheep which are not of this fold; I must bring them also, and they will hear My voice; and they will become one flock with one shepherd. For this reason the Father loves Me, because I lay down My life so that I may take it again. No one has taken it away from Me, but I lay it down on My own initiative. I have authority to lay it down,

and I have authority to take it up again. This commandment I received from My Father."

John 10:1–18

List all the promises from this chapter.

What is the abundant life?

_____

_____

_____

Who gives the abundant life?

_____

_____

_____

What does *door* refer to?

_____

_____

In your own words, from this portion of John, what
and who is Jesus?

_____

_____

_____

_____

How can we be saved?

_____

_____

_____

Who has the authority to allow us into heaven?

_____

_____

_____

_____

_____

_____

_____

Sing to the Lord a new song.
Praise God for who He is.
Give Him thanks for what He has done.

I am the true vine, and My Father is the vinedresser, Every branch in Me that does not bear fruit, He takes away; And every branch that bears fruit, He prunes it so that it bears more fruit. You are already clean because of the word which I have spoken to you. Abide in Me and I in you. As the *branch cannot bear fruit of itself unless it abides in the vine, so neither can you unless you abide in Me. I am the vine, you are the branches; he who abides in Me and I in him, he bears much fruit, for apart from Me you can do nothing.* If anyone does not abide in Me, he is thrown away and dries up; And they gather them, and cast them into the fire, and they are burned. *If you abide in Me and My words abide in you, ask whatever you wish, and it will be done for you. My Father is glorified by this, that you bear much fruit, and so prove to be My disciples. Just as the Father has loved Me, I have loved you; abide in My love. If you keep My commandments, you will abide in My love, just as I have kept my Father's commandments and abide in His love. These things I have spoken to you so that My joy may be in you and that your joy may be full. This is My commandment, that you love one another, just as I have loved you. Greater love has no one than this, that one lay down his life for his friends. You are My friends if you do what I command you.* He who hates Me, hates My Father also. If I had not done among them the works which no one else did, they would not have sin, but now they have both seen and hated Me and My Father as well. But they have done this to fulfill the word that is written in their Law, "They hated Me without cause." *When the Helper comes, whom I will send to you from the Father, that is the Spirit of truth who proceeds from the Father, He will testify about Me, and you will testify also, because you have been with Me from the beginning.*

John 15:1–14, 23–27

In your own words, what kind of fruit is John talking about?

_____

_____

_____

What does it mean to "abide in Me?"

_____

_____

_____

How do we abide?

_____

_____

_____

What does "Your fruit would remain" mean?

_____

_____

_____

Who is the Helper?

_____

_____

_____

Sing to the Lord a new song.
Praise God for who He is.
Give Him thanks for what He has done.

These things they will do because they have not
known the Father or Me. But these things I have
spoken to you, so that when their hour comes,
you may remember that I told you of them.
These things I did not say to you at the beginning, because I was with you. But now I am going
to Him who sent Me; and none of you ask Me,
"Where are you going?" But because I have said
these things to you, sorrow has filled your heart.
*But I tell you the truth, it is to your advantage that I
go away; for if I do not go away, the Helper will not
come to you; but if I go, I will send Him to you. And
He, when He comes, will convict the world concerning sin and righteousness and judgment; concerning
sin, because they do not believe in Me; and concerning righteousness, because I go to the Father and you
no longer see Me; and concerning judgment, because
the ruler of this world has been judged. I have many*

more things to say to you, but you cannot bear them now. But when He, the Spirit of Truth comes, He will guide you into all truth; for He will not speak on His own initiative, but whatever He hears, He will speak; and He will disclose to you what is to come. He will glorify Me, for He will take of Mine and will disclose it to you. All things that the Father has are Mine; therefore I said that He takes of Mine and will disclose it to you. A little while and you will no longer see Me, and again a little while, and you will see Me. Some of His disciples then said to one another, "What is this thing He is telling us, a little while, and you will not see Me, and again a little while, you will see Me; because I go to the Father?" So they were saying, "What is this that He says, "a little while? We do not know what He is talking about." Jesus knew that they wished to question Him, and He said to them, "Are you deliberating together about this, that I said, 'a little while, and you will not see Me, and again a little while, and you will see Me?' Truly, truly, I say to you, "that you will weep and lament, but your grief will be turned to joy. *These things I have spoken to you, so that in Me you may have peace. In the world you have tribulation, but take courage; I have overcome the world."*

John 16:3–33

How do we receive the spirit of truth?

_____

_____

What will the spirit of truth do for us?

_____

_____

_____

What does "overcome the world" mean to you?

_____

_____

_____

_____

How do we overcome the world?

_____

_____

_____

_____

_____

_____

_____

Where does true peace come from?

_____

_____

_____

How do we receive this kind of peace?

_____

_____

_____

Sing to the Lord a new song.
Praise God for who He is.
Give Him thanks for what He has done.

> Jesus spoke these things; and lifting His eyes to
> heaven, He said, "Father, the hour has come; glorify
> Your Son, that the Son may glorify You, even as You
> gave Him authority over all flesh, that to all whom
> You have given Him, He may give eternal life. This
> is eternal life, that they may know You, the only true
> God and Jesus Christ whom You have sent. I glorified
> You on earth, having accomplished the work which
> You have given Me to do. Now, Father, glorify Me

together with Yourself, with the glory which I had with You before the world was. I have manifested Your name to the men whom You gave Me out of the world; they were Yours and You gave them to Me and they have kept Your word. Now they have come to know that everything You have given Me is from You; for the words which You gave Me I have given to them; and they received them and truly understood that I came forth from You, and they believed that You sent Me. I ask on their behalf; I do not ask on behalf of the world, but of those You have given Me; for they are Yours; And Yours are Mine; and I have been glorified in them. I am no longer in the world; and yet they themselves are in the world, and I come to You, Holy Father, keep them in Your name, the name which You have given Me, that they may be one as We are. While I was with them I was keeping them in Your name which You have given Me; The glory which You have given Me I have given to them, that they may be one, just as We are one; I in them, and You in Me, that they may be per-fected in unity, so that the world may know that You sent Me, and loved them, even as You have loved Me. Father, I desire that they also whom You have given Me, be with Me where I am, so that they may see My glory which You have given Me, For You loved Me before the foundation of the world. O righteous Father, although the world has not known You; Yet I have known You; and these have known that You sent Me; And I have made Your name known to them, and will make it known so that the love which You loved Me may be in them, and I in them."

John 17

What is eternal life?

_____

_____

_____

List all the things Jesus prays for.

_____

_____

_____

List all the characteristics of Jesus.

_____

_____

_____

Who is the son of perdition?

_____

_____

_____

What is truth?

_____

_____

_____

If Jesus prays for us, would He not take care of us?

Sing to the Lord a new song.
Praise God for who He is.
Give Him thanks for what He has done.

> Now on the first day of the week Mary Magdalene came early to the tomb, while it was still dark, and saw the stone already taken away from the tomb. So she ran and came to Simon Peter and to the other disciple whom Jesus loved, and said to them, "They have taken away the Lord from the tomb, and we do not know where they have laid Him." So Peter and the other disciples went forth, and they were going to the tomb. The two were running together; and the other disciples ran ahead faster than Peter and came to the tomb first; and stooping and looking in, he saw the linen wrappings lying there; but did not go in. And so Simon Peter also came, following him, and entered the tomb; And he saw the linen wrappings lying there, and the face cloth which had been on His head, not lying with the linens wrappings, but rolled up in a place by itself. So the other disciples who had first come to the tomb then also entered, and *he saw and believed.* For as yet they did not understand the scripture, that He must rise again

from the dead. So the disciples went away to their homes. But Mary was standing outside the tomb; weeping; and so as she wept she stooped and looked into the tomb; And she saw two angels in white sitting, one at the head and one at the feet where the body of Jesus had been lying. And they said to her, "Woman, why are you weeping?" She said to them, "Because they have taken away my Lord, and I do not know where they have laid Him." When she had said this, she turned around and saw Jesus standing there, and did not know it was Jesus. Jesus said to her, "Woman, why are you weeping? Whom are you seeking?" Supposing Him to be a gardener, she said to Him, "Sir, if you have carried Him away, tell me where you have laid Him, and I will take Him away." Jesus said to her, "Mary!" She turned to Him and said to Him in Hebrew, *"Rabboni!" (which means teacher).* Jesus said to her, "Stop clinging to Me, for I have not yet ascended to the Father; but go to My brethren and say to them, 'I ascend to my Father and your Father, and My God and your God.'" Mary Magdalene came, announcing to the disciples, "I have seen the Lord," *"Peace be with you;* We have seen the Lord!" But he said to them, "Unless I see in His hands the imprint of the nails, and put my fingers into the place of the nails, and put my hand into His side, I will not believe." After eight days His disciples were again inside, and Thomas with them. Jesus came, the doors having been shut, and stood in their midst and said, "Peace be with you." Then He said to Thomas, "Reach here with your finger, and see My hands, and reach hear your hand and put it in My side; And do not be unbelieving, but believing." Thomas answered and said to Him, *"My Lord, my God! Blessed are they who did not see, and yet believed."* Therefore many other signs *Jesus also performed in the presence of the disciples, which are not written in this book; But these have been written so that you may believe that Jesus is the Christ, the Son of God; and that believing, you may have life in His name.*

John 20

In your own words, what happened in this portion of Scripture?

_____

_____

_____

Without the death, there would be no burial.
Without the burial, there would be no resurrection.
Without the resurrection, there would be no life "in His name."

Sing to the Lord a new song.
Praise God for who He is.
Give Him thanks for what He has done.

For I am not ashamed of the gospel, for it is the power of God for salvation to everyone who believes, to the Jews first and also to the Greek. For in it the righteousness of God is revealed from faith to faith; as it is written, "But the righteous man shall live by faith." For the wrath of God is revealed from heaven against all ungodliness and unrighteousness of men who suppress the truth in unrighteousness, Because that which is known about God is evident within them; for God made it evident to them. *For since the creation of the world His invisible attributes, His eternal power and divine nature, have been clearly seen* being understood through what has been made, so that *they are without excuse.* For even though they knew God, *they did not honor Him as God or give thanks,* but they became futile in their speculations, and their foolish heart was darkened. Professing to be wise, they became fools, and exchanged the glory of the incorruptible God for an image in the form of corruptible man and of birds and four-footed animals and crawling creatures. Therefore God gave them over in the lusts of their hearts to impurity, so that their bodies would be dishonored among them. For they exchanged the truth of God for a lie, and worshipped and served the creature rather than the Creator, who is blessed forever, amen. For this reason God gave them over to degrading passions; for their women exchanged the natural functions for that which is unnatural, and in the same way also men abandoned the natural function of the women and burned in their desire toward one another, men with men committing indecent acts and receiving in their own persons the due penalty of their error. And just as they did not see fit to acknowledge God any longer, God gave them over to a depraved mind, to do those things which are not proper, being filled with all unrighteousness, wickedness, greed, evil, full of envy, murder, strife, deceit, malice; they are gossips, slanders, haters of God, insolent, boastful, inventors of evil, disobe-

dient to parents, without understanding, untrust-
worthy, unloving, unmerciful, and although they
know the ordinance of God, that those who practice such things are worthy of death, they not only
do the same, but also give hearty approval to those
who practice them.

Romans 1:16–32

Define "invisible attributes, eternal power, and divine
nature."

_____

_____

_____

List all the attributes of God from Romans 1.

_____

_____

_____

What does the "glory of God" look like to you?

_____

_____

_____

What does "the righteous man lives by faith" mean to you?

_____

_____

_____

Sing to the Lord a new song.
Praise God for who He is.
Give Him thanks for what He has done.

What then? Are we better than they? Not at all; for we have already charged that both Jews and Greek are all under sin; as it is written,

"There is none righteous, not even one; There is none who understands,

There is none who seeks God; all have turned aside, together they have become useless; There is none who does good, There is not even one. 'Their throat is an open grave, With their tongues they keep deceiving, whose mouth is full of cursing and bitterness. "Their feet are swift to shed blood, Destruction and misery are in their paths, And the path of peace they have not known." "There is no fear of God before their eyes." Now we know what ever the Law says, it speaks to those under the Law, so that every mouth may be closed and *all the world may become accountable to God;* Because by the works of the Law no flesh will be justified in His sight; for through the Law comes knowledge of sin. *But now apart from the Law the righteousness of God has been manifested,* being witnessed by the Law and the Prophets, Even the righteousness of God through faith in Jesus Christ for all those who believe; *for there is no distinction, For all have sinned and fall short of the glory of God, Being justified as a gift by His grace through the redemption which is in Christ Jesus whom God displayed publicly as a propitiation in His blood through faith.* This was to demonstrate His righteousness, because in the forbearance of God He passed over the sins previously committed; For the demonstration, I say, of His righteousness at the present time, so that He would be the justifier of the one who has faith in Jesus.

Romans 3:9–26

Having read Romans 3, who do you say Jesus is?

_____

_____

_____

What are the characteristics of Jesus in Romans 3?

_____

_____

_____

What does Romans 3:23 say?

_____

_____

_____

What is the difference between the law and grace?

_____

_____

_____

Sing to the Lord a new song.
Praise God for who He is.
Give Him thanks for what He has done.

> For the promise to Abraham or to his descen-
> dents that he would be heir of the world *was not
> through the Law, but through the righteousness of
> faith.* For if those who are of the Law are heirs,
> faith is made void and the promise is nullified; for
> the Law brings about wrath, but where there is no
> Law, there also is no violation. *For this reason it is
> by faith, in order that it may be in accordance with
> grace, so that the promise will be guaranteed to all the
> descendants, not only be to those who are of the Law,
> but also to those who are of the faith* of Abraham,
> who is the father of us all, (as it is written, "A father
> of many nations have I made you") in the presence
> of him who believed, even God, who gives life to
> the dead and calls into being that which does not
> exist. *In hope against hope He believed,* so that He
> might become a father of many nations according
> to that which had been spoken. So shall all your

descendants be." Without becoming weak in faith he contemplated his own body, now as good as dead since he was about a hundred years old, and in the deadness of Sarah's womb; *Yet, with respect to the promise of God, he did not waver in unbelief but grew strong in faith, giving glory to God, and being fully assured that what God had promised, He was able also to perform.* Therefore it was also credited to him as righteousness. Now not for his sake only was it written that it was credited to him, but for our sake also, to whom it will be credited, as those who believe in Him who raised Jesus our Lord from the dead, He who was delivered over because of our transgressions, and was raised because of our justification.

Romans 4:13–25

What is faith?

_____

_____

_____

What is the promise?

_____

_____

_____

Define righteousness.

_____

_____

_____

What does *justification* mean?

_____

_____

_____

Sing to the Lord a new song.
Praise God for who He is.
Give Him thanks for what He has done.

> *Therefore, having been justified by faith, we have
> peace with God through our Lord Jesus Christ, through
> whom also we have obtained our introduction by
> faith into this grace in which we stand; and we exult
> in hope of the glory of God. And not only this, but we
> also exult in our tribulations, knowing that tribula-
> tions bring about perseverance, and perseverance,
> proven character; and proven character, hope; and hope
> does not disappoint, because the love of God has been
> poured out within our hearts through the Holy Spirit
> who was given to us. For while we were still helpless,
> at the right time Christ died for the ungodly.* For one
> will hardly die for a righteous man; though per-
> haps for the good man someone would dare even

to die. *But God demonstrates His own love toward us, in that while we were yet sinners, Christ died for us.* Much more then, having now been justified by His blood, we shall be saved from the wrath of God *through Him. For if while we were enemies we were reconciled to God through the death of His Son, much more, having been reconciled, we shall be saved by His life. And not only this, but we also exult in God though our Lord Jesus Christ, through whom we have now received the reconciliation. Therefore just as one man's sin entered into the world, and death through sin, and death spread to all men because all sinned, for until the law sin was in the world, but sin is not imputed when there is no law. Nevertheless death reigned from Adam until Moses, even over those who had not sinned in the likeness of the offense of Adam, who is the type of him who was to come. But the free gift is not like the transgression, for if by the transgression of the one the many died, much more did the grace of God and the gift by the grace of the one man, Jesus Christ, abound to the many.* The gift is not like that which came through the one who sinned, for on the one hand the judgment arose from one transgression resulting in condemnation, but on the other hand the free gift arose from many transgressions, resulting in justification. For if by the transgression of the one, death reigned through the one, much more those who receive the abundance of grace and of the gift of righteousness will reign in life through the one, Jesus Christ. So then as through one transgression there resulted condemnation to all men, even so through one act of righteousness there resulted justification of life to all men. For as through one man's disobedience the many were made sinners, even so through the obedience of the One man the many will be made righteous. The law came in so that the transgression would increase; but where sin increased, grace abounded all the more, so that as sin reigned in death *even so grace would reign through righteousness to eternal life through Jesus Christ our Lord.*

Romans 5

What does *reconciled* mean?

_____

_____

_____

_____

_____

What does it mean to have peace with God?

_____

_____

_____

What is the promise granted through faith in Jesus?

_____

_____

What is grace?

_____

_____

Sing to the Lord a new song.
Praise God for who He is.
Give Him thanks for what He has done.

What shall we say then? Are we to continue in sin
so that grace may increase? May it never be! How
shall we who died to sin live in it? Or do you not
know that all of us who have been baptized into
Christ Jesus have been baptized into His death?
Therefore we have been buried with Him through
baptism into death, so that as Christ was raised
from the dead through the glory of the Father,
so we too might walk in newness of life. *For if we
have become united with Him in the likeness of His
death, Certainly we shall also be in the likeness of His
resurrection, knowing this, our old self was crucified
with Him, in order that our body of sin might be done
away with, so that we would no longer be slaves to
sin; For he who has died is free from sin. Now if we
have died with Christ, we believe we shall also live
with Him, Knowing that Christ, having been raised
from the dead, is never to die again; Death no longer
is master over Him. For the death He died, He died
to sin once for all; but the life He lives, He lives to
God. Even so consider yourselves to be dead to sin,
but alive to God in Jesus Christ. Therefore do not let
sin reign in your mortal body so that you obey its lust,
And do not go on presenting the members of your body
to sin as instruments of unrighteousness; but pres-*

ent yourselves to God as those alive from the dead, and your members as instruments of righteousness to God. For sin shall not be master over you, for you are not under law, but under grace. What then, shall we sin because we are not under law but under grace? May it never be! Do you not know that when you present yourselves to someone as slaves to obedience, you are slaves to the one whom you obey, either sin resulting in death, or of obedience resulting in righteousness? But *thanks be to God* that though you were slaves of sin, you became *obedient from the heart* to that form of teaching to which you were committed, and having been freed from sin, you became slaves of righteousness For the outcome of those things is death. But now having been freed from sin and enslaved to God, you derive your benefit, resulting in sanctification, and the outcome, eternal life. *For the wages of sin is death, but the free gift of God is eternal life in Jesus Christ our Lord.*

Romans 6

What allows us to be free from sin?

_____

_____

_____

How are we alive to God?

_____

_____

_____

_____

What does *sanctification* mean?

_____

_____

How do we receive eternal life?

_____

_____

_____

Sing to the Lord a new song.
Praise God for who He is.
Give Him thanks for what He has done.

> *Therefore, my brethren, you also were made to die to the Law through the body of Christ, so that you might be joined to another, to Him who was raised from the dead, in order that we might bear fruit for God.* For while we were in the flesh, the sinful passions, which were aroused by the Law, were at work in our body to bear fruit for death. But now we have been released from the Law, having died to that by which we were bound, so that we serve in *newness of Spirit* and not in oldness of the letter. What

shall we say then? Is the Law sin? May it never be! On the contrary, I would not have come to know sin except through the Law; for I would not have known about coveting if the Law had not said, "You shall not covet." But sin, taking opportunity through the commandment, produced in me coveting of every kind; for apart from the Law sin is dead. I was once alive apart from the Law; but when the commandment came, sin became alive and I died; and this commandment, which was to result in life, proved to result in death for me; For sin, taking an opportunity through the commandment, deceived me and through it killed me. So then, the Law is holy, and the commandment is holy and righteous and good. Therefore did that which is good become a cause of death for me? May it never be! Rather it was sin in order that it might be shown to be sin by affecting my death through that which is good, so that through the commandment sin would be utterly sinful. For we know that the Law is spiritual, but I am of the flesh, sold into bondage to sin. For what I am doing I do not understand; for I am not practicing what I would like to do, but I am doing the very thing I hate. But if I do the very thing I do not want to do, I agree with the law, confessing that the law is good. So now, no longer am I the one doing it, but sin which dwells in me. For I know that nothing good dwells in me, that is, in my flesh; for the willing is present in me, but the doing of good is not. For the good that I want, I do not do, but I practice the very evil that I do not want, But if I am doing the very thing I do not want, I am no longer the one doing it, but sin which dwells in me. I find then that evil is present in me, the one who wants to do good. *For I joy-fully concur with the Law of God, in the inner man, But I see a different law in the members of my body, waging war against the law of my mind and making me a prisoner of the law of sin which is in my members.* Wretched man that I am! Who will set me free from the body of this death? *Thanks be to Jesus Christ our Lord!* So then, on one hand I myself with my mind am serving the Law of God, but on the other, with my flesh the law of sin.

Romans 7:4–25

What are the principles of God?

_____

_____

_____

How do we overcome sin?

_____

_____

_____

Who is God?

_____

_____

_____

_____

What is the war between the mind and the flesh?

_____

_____

_____

_____

_____

Sing to the Lord a new song.
Praise God for who He is.
Give Him thanks for what He has done.

> *Therefore there is now no condemnation for those who are in Christ Jesus. For the law of the Spirit of life in Christ Jesus has set you free from the law of sin and death.* For what the Law could not do weak as it was through the flesh, God did; sending His own Son in the likeness of sinful flesh and as an offering for sin, He condemned sin in the flesh, so that the requirement of the Law might be fulfilled in us, who do not walk according to the flesh but according to the Spirit. *For those who walk accord-*

ing to the flesh set their mind of the flesh, but those who walk according to the Spirit, the things of the Spirit. For the mind set on the flesh is death, but the *mind set on the Spirit is life and peace,* because the mind set on the flesh is hostile toward God; for it does not subject itself to the Law of God, for it is not even able to do so, and those who are in the flesh cannot please God. However, you are not in the flesh but in the Spirit, if indeed the Spirit of God dwells in you, But if anyone who does not have the Spirit of Christ, he does not belong to Him. If Christ is in you, though the body is dead because of sin, *yet the Spirit is alive because of righteousness.* But if the Spirit of Him who raised Jesus from the dead dwells in you, He who raised Christ Jesus from the dead will also give life to your mortal bodies through His Spirit who dwells in you. So then, brethren, we are under obligation, not to the flesh, to live according to the flesh-for if we are living according to the flesh, you must die; but if by the Spirit you are putting to death the deeds of the body, you will live. For all who are being led by the Spirit of God, are the sons of God. For you have not received a Spirit of slavery leading to fear again, but you received a Spirit of adoption as sons by which we cry out "Abba father!" The Spirit Himself testifies with our spirit that we are children of God, and if children, heirs also, heirs of God and *fellow heirs with Christ, if indeed we suffer with Him so that we may also be glorified with Him. For I consider that the suffering of the present time are not worthy to be compared with the glory that is to be revealed to us.* And not only this, but also we ourselves, having the first fruits of the Spirit, even we ourselves groan within ourselves, waiting eagerly for our adoption as sons, the redemption of our body. For in hope we have been saved, but hope that is seen is not hope; for who hopes for what he already sees? But if we hope for what we do not see, *with perseverance we wait eagerly for it.* In the same way the Spirit also helps our weakness; for we do not know how to pray as we should, but the Spirit Himself intercedes for us with groanings too deep for words; And He who searches the hearts knows what the mind of the Spirit is, because He intercedes for the saints according to the will of God. *And we know that God causes all things to work out for good to those who love God, to those who are called according to His purpose.* For those whom He foreknew, He also predestined to become conformed to the image of His Son, so that He would be the firstborn among many brethren; and these whom He predestined, He also called; And these whom He called, He also justified; and these whom He justified, He also glorified. What then shall we say, If God is for us, who can be against us? He who did not spare His own Son, but delivered Him over for us all, how will He not also with Him freely give us all things? Who will bring a charge against God's elect? God is the one who justifies; Who is the one who condemns? Christ Jesus is the one who died, yes rather the one who was raised from the dead, who is at the right hand of God, who also intercedes for us. Who *will separate us from the love of Christ? Will tribulation, or distress, or persecution, or famine, or nakedness, or peril, or sword? Just as it is written: We are being put to death all day long;*

We are to be considered as sheep to be slaughtered."

But in all these things we overwhelmingly con-quer through Him who loved us. For I am convinced

*that neither death, nor life, nor angels, nor princi-
palities nor things to come, nor powers, nor height,
nor depth, nor any other created thing, will be able
to separate us from the love of God which is in Christ
Jesus.*

Romans 8

What do these words mean to you in reference to this scripture?

1. "predestined"
2. "called"
3. "justified"
4. "glorified"

What is our position through the Spirit of God?

_____

_____

_____

Who or what can separate us from life with Jesus?

_____

_____

_____

What are we in Jesus?

_____

_____

_____

_____

Sing to the Lord a new song.
Praise God for who He is.
Give Him thanks for what He has done.

> *Therefore I urge you, brethren, by the mercies of God,*
> *present your bodies a living and holy sacrifice, accept-*
> *able to God, which is your spiritual service of wor-*
> *ship. And do not be conformed to this world, but be*
> *transformed by the renewing of your mind, so that*
> *you may prove what the will of God is, that which*
> *is good and acceptable and perfect.* For through the
> grace given to me I say to everyone among you not
> to think more highly of himself than he ought to
> think; but to think so as to have sound judgment,
> as God has allotted to each a measure of faith. For
> just as we have many members in one body and
> all the members do not have the same function,
> So we, who are many, are one body in Christ, and
> individually members of one another. Do not be
> overcome by evil, but overcome evil with good.
>
> Romans 12

What are the mercies of God?

_____

_____

What is good and acceptable to God?

_____

_____

_____

What does renewing your mind mean?

_____

_____

_____

Why the mind?

_____

_____

_____

What is grace?

_____

_____

_____

_____

Sing to the Lord a new song.
Praise God for who He is.
Give Him thanks for what He has done.

> Now *I make known to you, brethren, the gospel which I preached to you, which also you received, in which also you stand, By which also you are saved, if you hold fast the word which I preached to you, unless you believed in vain.* Now if Christ is preached, that He has been raised from the dead, how do some among you say that there is no resurrection of the dead? But if there is no resurrection of the dead, not even Christ has been raised; and if Christ has not been raised, then our preaching is vain, your faith also is vain. Moreover we are even found to be false witnesses of God, because we testified against God that He raised Christ, whom He did not raise, if in fact the dead are not raised. For if the dead are not raised, not even Christ has been raised, your faith is worthless; you are still in your sins. Then those who have fallen asleep in Christ have perished. If we have hoped in Christ in this life only, we are all men most to be pitied. But now Christ has been risen from the dead, the first fruits of those who are asleep. For since by a man came death, by a Man also came the resurrection of the dead. For as in Adam all die, so also in Christ all will be made alive. But each in his own order; Christ the first fruits, after that those who are Christ at His coming, then comes the end, when He hands over the kingdom to the God and Father, when He has abolished all rule and all authority and power. For He must reign until He has put all His enemies under His feet. The last enemy that will be abolished is death.

For He has put all things in subjection under His feet. But when He says, "All things are put in subjection," it is evident that He is excepted who put all things in subjection to Him. There are also heavenly bodies and earthly bodies, but the glory of the heavenly is one and the glory of the earthly is another. There is one glory of the sun, and another of the moon, and another glory of the stars; for star differs from star in glory. So also is the resurrection of the dead. It is sown a perishable body, it is raised an imperishable body; It is sown in dishonor, it is raised in glory; it is sown in weakness, it is raised in power; It is sown a natural body, it is raised a spiritual body. If there is a natural body, there is also a spiritual body. So also it is written, "The first man Adam became a living soul." The last Adam became a life giving spirit. However, the spiritual is not first, but the natural, then the spiritual. The first man is from the earth, earthy; the second man is from heaven. As is the earthy, so also are those who are earthy; and as is the heavenly, so also are those who are heavenly. Just as we have borne the image of the earthy, we also bear the image of the heavenly. Now I say this, brethren, that flesh and blood cannot inherit the kingdom of God; nor does the perishable inherit the imperishable. Behold I tell you a mystery; we will not all sleep, but we will all be changed, in a moment, in the twinkling of an eye, at the last trumpet; for the trumpet will sound, and the dead will be raised imperishable, and we will be changed. For this perishable must put on the imperishable, and this mortal will have put on immortality. Then will come about the saying that is written, "Death is swallowed in victory, O death where is your victory? O death where is your sting?" The sting of death is sin, and the power of sin is the law; *but thanks be to God, who gives us the victory in our Lord Jesus Christ. Therefore, my beloved brethren, be steadfast, immovable, always abounding in the work of the Lord, knowing that your toil is not in vain in the Lord.*

1 Corinthians 15:1–2, 12–27, 40–58

Paraphrase this scripture in your own words.

_____

_____

_____

What does it mean to die daily?

_____

_____

_____

What is the difference between the earthly and heavenly body?

_____

_____

_____

What is the final victory?

_____

_____

_____

How can we have victory?

_____

_____

_____

Sing to the Lord a new song.
Praise God for who He is.
Give Him thanks for what He has done.

> Blessed be the God and Father of our *Lord Jesus Christ who has blessed us with every spiritual blessing in the heavenly places in Christ,* just as He chose us in Him before the foundation of the world, that we would be holy and blameless before Him. In love He predestined us to adoption as sons through Jesus Christ to Himself, according to the kind intention of His will, to the praise of the glory of His grace, which He freely bestowed on us in the beloved. In Him we have redemption through His blood, the forgiveness of our trespass, according to the riches of His grace, which He lavished on us in all wisdom and insight. *He made known to us the mystery of His* will, according to His

kind intention which He purposed in Him with a *view to an administration suitable to the fullness of the times, that is, the summing up of all things in Christ, things in the heavens and things on the earth. In Him also we have obtained an inheritance, having been predestined according to His purpose who works all things after the counsel of His will, to the end that we who are the first to hope in Christ would be to the praise of His glory. In Him, you also, after listening to the message of truth, the gospel of your salvation, having also believed, you were sealed in Him with the Holy Spirit of promise, Who is given as a pledge of our inheritance, with a view to the redemption of God's own possession, to the praise of His glory.*

Ephesians 1:3–14

What does "have been blessed with every spiritual blessing" mean?

_____

_____

_____

What is the mystery of God's will?

List all of God's characteristics from this scripture.

_____

_____

_____

What has God done for us?

_____

_____

_____

What has God given us?

_____

_____

_____

God's will for us is found in Ephesians 1:12: "That we who were the first to hope in Christ Jesus would be to the praise of His glory." What does it mean to be the "praise of His glory?

Sing to the Lord a new song.
Praise God for who He is.
Give Him thanks for what He has done.

_____

_____

_____

I hope and pray after you have read this book, you understand and experience the transforming power of who God really is in all His grace, mercy, strength, power, and loving kindness. May you be able to see His nature and character at work in your own life and be able to "sing to Him a new song," give Him praise for who He really is, and thank Him for what He has done!

Yes I am boasting in the Lord! Jeremiah 9:24: "Let him who boasts boast of this, that he understands and knows Me, that I am the Lord who exercises loving kindness, justice, righteousness on the earth; for I delight in these things, declares the Lord."